THIS BOOK BELONGS TO

NAME
ADDRESS

EMAIL
PHONE

EMERGENCY CONTACT 1

NAME
PHONE

EMERGENCY CONTACT 2

NAME
PHONE

This book is not intended as a substitute for the medical advice of physicians. The reader should regularly consult a physician in matters relating to his/her health and particularly with respect to any symptoms that may require diagnosis or medical attention.

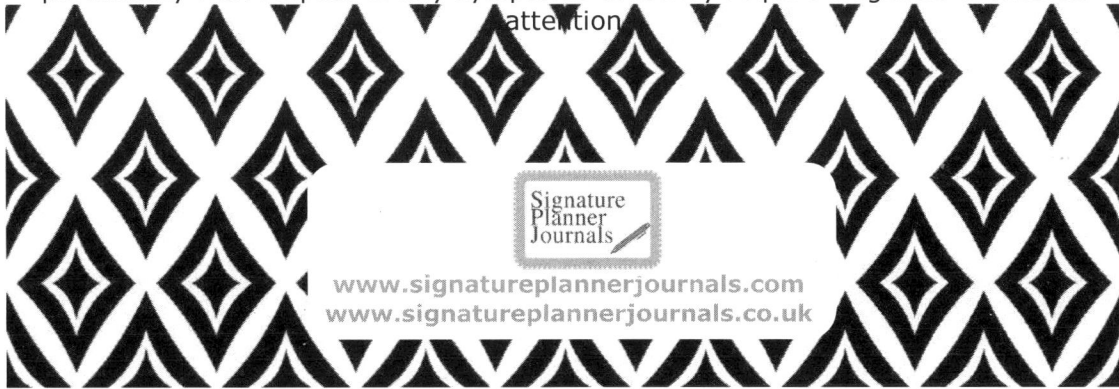

Signature Planner Journals

www.signatureplannerjournals.com
www.signatureplannerjournals.co.uk

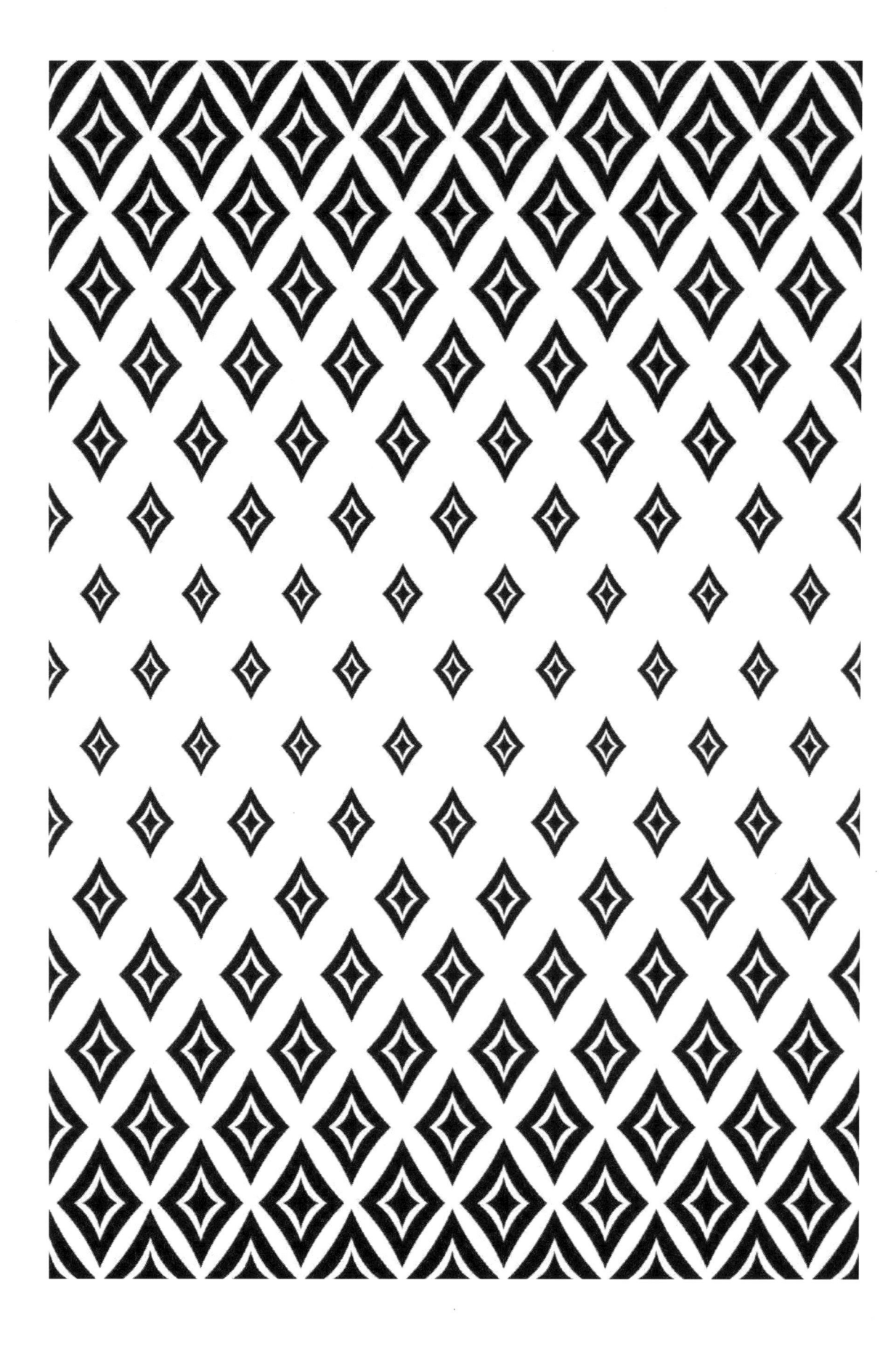

CONTENTS

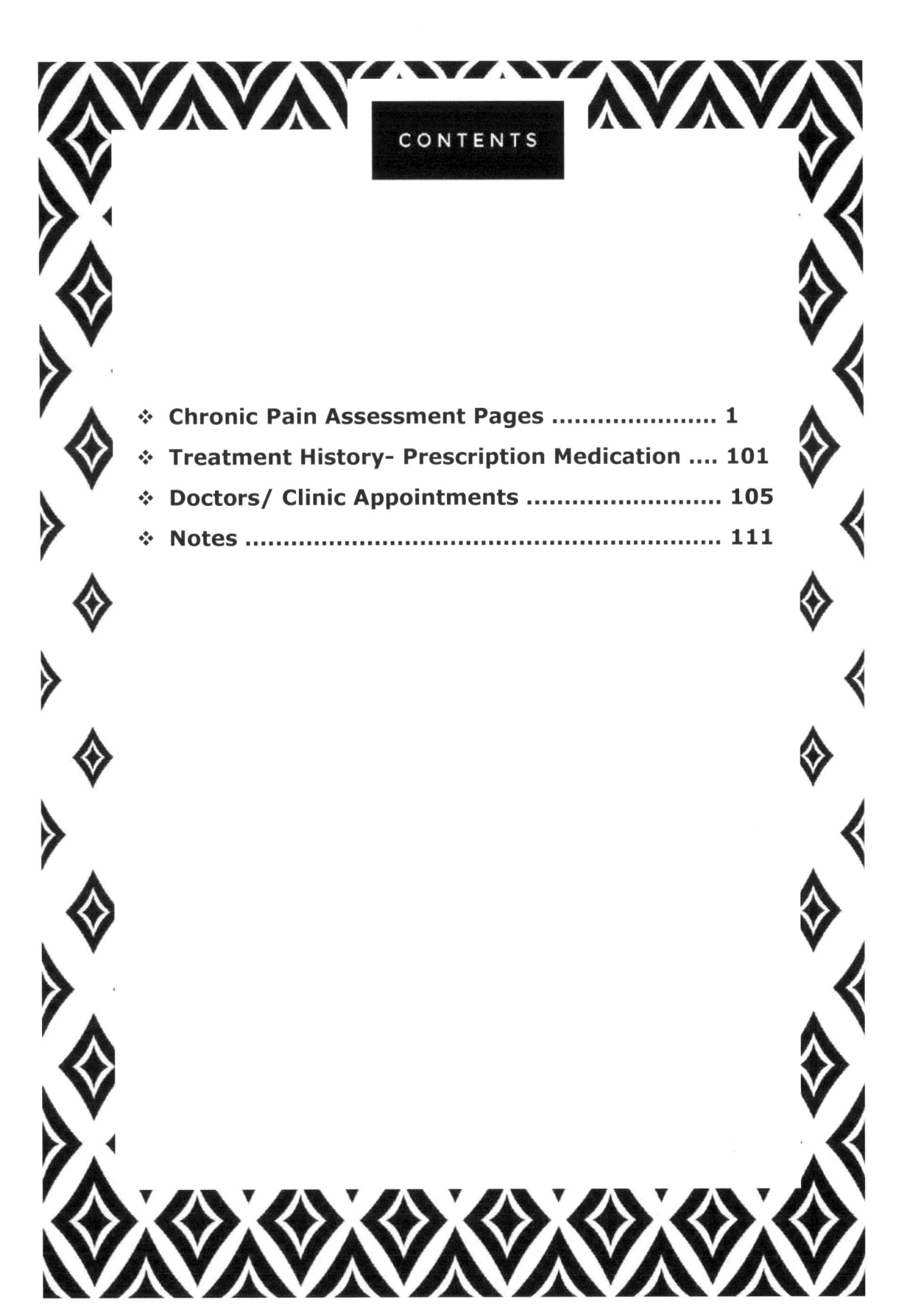

- ❖ **Chronic Pain Assessment Pages** 1
- ❖ **Treatment History- Prescription Medication** 101
- ❖ **Doctors/ Clinic Appointments** 105
- ❖ **Notes** 111

CHRONIC PAIN ASSESSMENT

DATE		DAY	
TIME STARTED		TIME ENDED	
TOTAL DURATION			

← Mark the location of the pain

LENGTH OF TIME EXPERIENCING THE PAIN?

< 6 Months		6-12 Months	
1-3 Years		3 Years +	

TYPE OF PAIN

Indescribable		Stabbing		Sharp	
Burning		Aching		Prickly	
Numb		Tingling/ Pins & Needles			
Other					

EXTERNAL ENVIROMENTAL FACTORS

Sun/ Heat		Cold		Windy	
Rain		Aching		Cloudy	
Other					

PAIN SCALE
NO PAIN ⟶ SEVERE PAIN

0	1	2	3	4	5	6	7	8	9	10

SUSPECTED TRIGGERS

-
-
-
-

-
-
-
-

SYMPTOMS

RELIEF MEASURES

NOTES

CHRONIC PAIN ASSESSMENT

DATE		DAY	
TIME STARTED		TIME ENDED	
TOTAL DURATION			

RIGHT SIDE BACK FRONT LEFT SIDE

⬅ Mark the location of the pain

LENGTH OF TIME EXPERIENCING THE PAIN?

< 6 Months		6-12 Months	
1-3 Years		3 Years +	

TYPE OF PAIN

Indescribable		Stabbing		Sharp	
Burning		Aching		Prickly	
Numb		Tingling/ Pins & Needles			
Other					

EXTERNAL ENVIROMENTAL FACTORS

Sun/ Heat		Cold		Windy	
Rain		Aching		Cloudy	
Other					

PAIN SCALE
NO PAIN ⟶ SEVERE PAIN

0	1	2	3	4	5	6	7	8	9	10

SUSPECTED TRIGGERS
-
-
-
-
-
-
-
-

SYMPTOMS

RELIEF MEASURES

NOTES

CHRONIC PAIN ASSESSMENT

DATE		DAY	
TIME STARTED		TIME ENDED	
TOTAL DURATION			

← Mark the location of the pain

LENGTH OF TIME EXPERIENCING THE PAIN?

< 6 Months		6-12 Months	
1-3 Years		3 Years +	

TYPE OF PAIN

Indescribable		Stabbing		Sharp	
Burning		Aching		Prickly	
Numb		Tingling/ Pins & Needles			
Other					

EXTERNAL ENVIROMENTAL FACTORS

Sun/ Heat		Cold		Windy	
Rain		Aching		Cloudy	
Other					

PAIN SCALE
NO PAIN ⎯⎯⎯⎯⎯⎯⎯⎯⎯⎯⎯⎯⎯⎯→ SEVERE PAIN

0	1	2	3	4	5	6	7	8	9	10

SUSPECTED TRIGGERS
-
-
-
-

SYMPTOMS

RELIEF MEASURES

NOTES

CHRONIC PAIN ASSESSMENT

DATE		DAY	
TIME STARTED		TIME ENDED	
TOTAL DURATION			

RIGHT SIDE BACK FRONT LEFT SIDE

⬅ Mark the location of the pain

LENGTH OF TIME EXPERIENCING THE PAIN?

< 6 Months		6-12 Months	
1-3 Years		3 Years +	

TYPE OF PAIN

Indescribable		Stabbing		Sharp	
Burning		Aching		Prickly	
Numb		Tingling/ Pins & Needles			
Other					

EXTERNAL ENVIROMENTAL FACTORS

Sun/ Heat		Cold		Windy	
Rain		Aching		Cloudy	
Other					

PAIN SCALE

NO PAIN ⟶ SEVERE PAIN

0	1	2	3	4	5	6	7	8	9	10

SUSPECTED TRIGGERS

-
-
-
-
-
-
-
-

SYMPTOMS

RELIEF MEASURES

NOTES

CHRONIC PAIN ASSESSMENT

DATE		DAY	
TIME STARTED		TIME ENDED	
TOTAL DURATION			

Mark the location of the pain

LENGTH OF TIME EXPERIENCING THE PAIN?

< 6 Months		6-12 Months	
1-3 Years		3 Years +	

TYPE OF PAIN

Indescribable		Stabbing		Sharp	
Burning		Aching		Prickly	
Numb		Tingling/ Pins & Needles			
Other					

EXTERNAL ENVIROMENTAL FACTORS

Sun/ Heat		Cold		Windy	
Rain		Aching		Cloudy	
Other					

PAIN SCALE
NO PAIN ⟶ SEVERE PAIN

0	1	2	3	4	5	6	7	8	9	10

SUSPECTED TRIGGERS

-
-
-
-

-
-
-
-

SYMPTOMS

RELIEF MEASURES

NOTES

CHRONIC PAIN ASSESSMENT

DATE		DAY	
TIME STARTED		TIME ENDED	
TOTAL DURATION			

← Mark the location of the pain

LENGTH OF TIME EXPERIENCING THE PAIN?

< 6 Months		6-12 Months	
1-3 Years		3 Years +	

TYPE OF PAIN

Indescribable		Stabbing		Sharp	
Burning		Aching		Prickly	
Numb		Tingling/ Pins & Needles			
Other					

EXTERNAL ENVIROMENTAL FACTORS

Sun/ Heat		Cold		Windy	
Rain		Aching		Cloudy	
Other					

PAIN SCALE
NO PAIN ⟶ SEVERE PAIN

0	1	2	3	4	5	6	7	8	9	10

SUSPECTED TRIGGERS
-
-
-
-
-
-
-
-

SYMPTOMS

RELIEF MEASURES

NOTES

CHRONIC PAIN ASSESSMENT

DATE		DAY	
TIME STARTED		TIME ENDED	
TOTAL DURATION			

← Mark the location of the pain

LENGTH OF TIME EXPERIENCING THE PAIN?

< 6 Months		6-12 Months	
1-3 Years		3 Years +	

TYPE OF PAIN

Indescribable		Stabbing		Sharp	
Burning		Aching		Prickly	
Numb		Tingling/ Pins & Needles			
Other					

EXTERNAL ENVIROMENTAL FACTORS

Sun/ Heat		Cold		Windy	
Rain		Aching		Cloudy	
Other					

PAIN SCALE
NO PAIN ─────────────────────→ SEVERE PAIN

0	1	2	3	4	5	6	7	8	9	10

SUSPECTED TRIGGERS

-
-
-
-

-
-
-
-

SYMPTOMS

RELIEF MEASURES

NOTES

CHRONIC PAIN ASSESSMENT

DATE		DAY	
TIME STARTED		TIME ENDED	
TOTAL DURATION			

RIGHT SIDE BACK FRONT LEFT SIDE

← Mark the location of the pain

LENGTH OF TIME EXPERIENCING THE PAIN?

< 6 Months		6-12 Months	
1-3 Years		3 Years +	

TYPE OF PAIN

Indescribable		Stabbing		Sharp	
Burning		Aching		Prickly	
Numb		Tingling/ Pins & Needles			
Other					

EXTERNAL ENVIROMENTAL FACTORS

Sun/ Heat		Cold		Windy	
Rain		Aching		Cloudy	
Other					

PAIN SCALE
NO PAIN ──────────────→ SEVERE PAIN

0	1	2	3	4	5	6	7	8	9	10

SUSPECTED TRIGGERS
-
-
-
-

-
-
-
-

SYMPTOMS

RELIEF MEASURES

NOTES

CHRONIC PAIN ASSESSMENT

DATE		DAY	
TIME STARTED		TIME ENDED	
TOTAL DURATION			

Mark the location of the pain

LENGTH OF TIME EXPERIENCING THE PAIN?

< 6 Months		6-12 Months	
1-3 Years		3 Years +	

TYPE OF PAIN

Indescribable		Stabbing		Sharp	
Burning		Aching		Prickly	
Numb		Tingling/ Pins & Needles			
Other					

EXTERNAL ENVIROMENTAL FACTORS

Sun/ Heat		Cold		Windy	
Rain		Aching		Cloudy	
Other					

PAIN SCALE
NO PAIN ⟶ SEVERE PAIN

0	1	2	3	4	5	6	7	8	9	10

SUSPECTED TRIGGERS

-
-
-
-

-
-
-
-

SYMPTOMS

RELIEF MEASURES

NOTES

CHRONIC PAIN ASSESSMENT

DATE		DAY	
TIME STARTED		TIME ENDED	
TOTAL DURATION			

RIGHT SIDE   BACK   FRONT   LEFT SIDE

⬅ Mark the location of the pain

LENGTH OF TIME EXPERIENCING THE PAIN?

< 6 Months		6-12 Months	
1-3 Years		3 Years +	

TYPE OF PAIN

Indescribable		Stabbing		Sharp	
Burning		Aching		Prickly	
Numb		Tingling/ Pins & Needles			
Other					

EXTERNAL ENVIROMENTAL FACTORS

Sun/ Heat		Cold		Windy	
Rain		Aching		Cloudy	
Other					

PAIN SCALE

NO PAIN ——————————————➡ SEVERE PAIN

0	1	2	3	4	5	6	7	8	9	10

SUSPECTED TRIGGERS

-
-
-
-
-
-
-
-

SYMPTOMS

_____
_____
_____
_____
_____
_____
_____

RELIEF MEASURES

_____
_____
_____
_____
_____
_____

NOTES

_____
_____
_____
_____
_____

CHRONIC PAIN ASSESSMENT

DATE		DAY	
TIME STARTED		TIME ENDED	
TOTAL DURATION			

Mark the location of the pain

LENGTH OF TIME EXPERIENCING THE PAIN?

< 6 Months		6-12 Months	
1-3 Years		3 Years +	

TYPE OF PAIN

Indescribable		Stabbing		Sharp	
Burning		Aching		Prickly	
Numb		Tingling/ Pins & Needles			
Other					

EXTERNAL ENVIROMENTAL FACTORS

Sun/ Heat		Cold		Windy	
Rain		Aching		Cloudy	
Other					

PAIN SCALE
NO PAIN ⟶ SEVERE PAIN

0	1	2	3	4	5	6	7	8	9	10

SUSPECTED TRIGGERS
-
-
-
-

SYMPTOMS

RELIEF MEASURES

NOTES

CHRONIC PAIN ASSESSMENT

DATE		DAY	
TIME STARTED		TIME ENDED	
TOTAL DURATION			

Mark the location of the pain

LENGTH OF TIME EXPERIENCING THE PAIN?
< 6 Months		6-12 Months	
1-3 Years		3 Years +	

TYPE OF PAIN
Indescribable		Stabbing		Sharp	
Burning		Aching		Prickly	
Numb		Tingling/ Pins & Needles			
Other					

EXTERNAL ENVIROMENTAL FACTORS
Sun/ Heat		Cold		Windy	
Rain		Aching		Cloudy	
Other					

PAIN SCALE
NO PAIN ⟶ SEVERE PAIN

0	1	2	3	4	5	6	7	8	9	10

SUSPECTED TRIGGERS
-
-
-
-
-
-
-
-

SYMPTOMS

RELIEF MEASURES

NOTES

CHRONIC PAIN ASSESSMENT

DATE		DAY	
TIME STARTED		TIME ENDED	
TOTAL DURATION			

Mark the location of the pain

LENGTH OF TIME EXPERIENCING THE PAIN?
< 6 Months		6-12 Months	
1-3 Years		3 Years +	

TYPE OF PAIN
Indescribable		Stabbing		Sharp	
Burning		Aching		Prickly	
Numb		Tingling/ Pins & Needles			
Other					

EXTERNAL ENVIROMENTAL FACTORS
Sun/ Heat		Cold		Windy	
Rain		Aching		Cloudy	
Other					

PAIN SCALE
NO PAIN ⟶ SEVERE PAIN

0	1	2	3	4	5	6	7	8	9	10

SUSPECTED TRIGGERS
-
-
-
-

-
-
-
-

SYMPTOMS

RELIEF MEASURES

NOTES

CHRONIC PAIN ASSESSMENT

DATE		DAY	
TIME STARTED		TIME ENDED	
TOTAL DURATION			

Mark the location of the pain

LENGTH OF TIME EXPERIENCING THE PAIN?

< 6 Months		6-12 Months	
1-3 Years		3 Years +	

TYPE OF PAIN

Indescribable		Stabbing		Sharp	
Burning		Aching		Prickly	
Numb		Tingling/ Pins & Needles			
Other					

EXTERNAL ENVIROMENTAL FACTORS

Sun/ Heat		Cold		Windy	
Rain		Aching		Cloudy	
Other					

PAIN SCALE

NO PAIN ──────────────────────────→ SEVERE PAIN

0	1	2	3	4	5	6	7	8	9	10

SUSPECTED TRIGGERS

-
-
-
-
-
-
-
-

SYMPTOMS

RELIEF MEASURES

NOTES

CHRONIC PAIN ASSESSMENT

DATE		DAY	
TIME STARTED		TIME ENDED	
TOTAL DURATION			

Mark the location of the pain

LENGTH OF TIME EXPERIENCING THE PAIN?

< 6 Months		6-12 Months	
1-3 Years		3 Years +	

TYPE OF PAIN

Indescribable		Stabbing		Sharp	
Burning		Aching		Prickly	
Numb		Tingling/ Pins & Needles			
Other					

EXTERNAL ENVIROMENTAL FACTORS

Sun/ Heat		Cold		Windy	
Rain		Aching		Cloudy	
Other					

PAIN SCALE
NO PAIN ──────────────────────────────→ SEVERE PAIN

0	1	2	3	4	5	6	7	8	9	10

SUSPECTED TRIGGERS
-
-
-
-

SYMPTOMS

RELIEF MEASURES

NOTES

CHRONIC PAIN ASSESSMENT

DATE		DAY	
TIME STARTED		TIME ENDED	
TOTAL DURATION			

Mark the location of the pain

LENGTH OF TIME EXPERIENCING THE PAIN?

< 6 Months		6-12 Months
1-3 Years		3 Years +

TYPE OF PAIN

Indescribable	Stabbing	Sharp
Burning	Aching	Prickly
Numb	Tingling/ Pins & Needles	
Other		

EXTERNAL ENVIROMENTAL FACTORS

Sun/ Heat	Cold	Windy
Rain	Aching	Cloudy
Other		

PAIN SCALE

NO PAIN ⟶ SEVERE PAIN

0	1	2	3	4	5	6	7	8	9	10

SUSPECTED TRIGGERS

-
-
-
-
-
-
-
-

SYMPTOMS

RELIEF MEASURES

NOTES

CHRONIC PAIN ASSESSMENT

DATE		DAY	
TIME STARTED		TIME ENDED	
TOTAL DURATION			

Mark the location of the pain

LENGTH OF TIME EXPERIENCING THE PAIN?

< 6 Months		6-12 Months	
1-3 Years		3 Years +	

TYPE OF PAIN

Indescribable		Stabbing		Sharp	
Burning		Aching		Prickly	
Numb		Tingling/ Pins & Needles			
Other					

EXTERNAL ENVIROMENTAL FACTORS

Sun/ Heat		Cold		Windy	
Rain		Aching		Cloudy	
Other					

PAIN SCALE
NO PAIN ⟶ SEVERE PAIN

0	1	2	3	4	5	6	7	8	9	10

SUSPECTED TRIGGERS

-
-
-
-

-
-
-
-

SYMPTOMS

RELIEF MEASURES

NOTES

CHRONIC PAIN ASSESSMENT

DATE		DAY	
TIME STARTED		TIME ENDED	
TOTAL DURATION			

Mark the location of the pain

LENGTH OF TIME EXPERIENCING THE PAIN?
< 6 Months		6-12 Months	
1-3 Years		3 Years +	

TYPE OF PAIN
Indescribable		Stabbing		Sharp	
Burning		Aching		Prickly	
Numb		Tingling/ Pins & Needles			
Other					

EXTERNAL ENVIROMENTAL FACTORS
Sun/ Heat		Cold		Windy	
Rain		Aching		Cloudy	
Other					

PAIN SCALE
NO PAIN ⟶ SEVERE PAIN

0	1	2	3	4	5	6	7	8	9	10

SUSPECTED TRIGGERS
-
-
-
-
-
-
-
-

SYMPTOMS

RELIEF MEASURES

NOTES

CHRONIC PAIN ASSESSMENT

DATE		DAY	
TIME STARTED		TIME ENDED	
TOTAL DURATION			

Mark the location of the pain

LENGTH OF TIME EXPERIENCING THE PAIN?

< 6 Months		6-12 Months	
1-3 Years		3 Years +	

TYPE OF PAIN

Indescribable		Stabbing		Sharp	
Burning		Aching		Prickly	
Numb		Tingling/ Pins & Needles			
Other					

EXTERNAL ENVIROMENTAL FACTORS

Sun/ Heat		Cold		Windy	
Rain		Aching		Cloudy	
Other					

PAIN SCALE
NO PAIN ──────────────────────────► SEVERE PAIN

0	1	2	3	4	5	6	7	8	9	10

SUSPECTED TRIGGERS

-
-
-
-

-
-
-
-

SYMPTOMS

RELIEF MEASURES

NOTES

CHRONIC PAIN ASSESSMENT

DATE		DAY	
TIME STARTED		TIME ENDED	
TOTAL DURATION			

Mark the location of the pain

LENGTH OF TIME EXPERIENCING THE PAIN?

< 6 Months		6-12 Months	
1-3 Years		3 Years +	

TYPE OF PAIN

Indescribable		Stabbing		Sharp	
Burning		Aching		Prickly	
Numb		Tingling/ Pins & Needles			
Other					

EXTERNAL ENVIROMENTAL FACTORS

Sun/ Heat		Cold		Windy	
Rain		Aching		Cloudy	
Other					

PAIN SCALE

NO PAIN ──────────────────────────→ SEVERE PAIN

0	1	2	3	4	5	6	7	8	9	10

SUSPECTED TRIGGERS

-
-
-
-

SYMPTOMS

RELIEF MEASURES

NOTES

CHRONIC PAIN ASSESSMENT

DATE		DAY	
TIME STARTED		TIME ENDED	
TOTAL DURATION			

← Mark the location of the pain

LENGTH OF TIME EXPERIENCING THE PAIN?

< 6 Months		6-12 Months	
1-3 Years		3 Years +	

TYPE OF PAIN

Indescribable		Stabbing		Sharp	
Burning		Aching		Prickly	
Numb		Tingling/ Pins & Needles			
Other					

EXTERNAL ENVIROMENTAL FACTORS

Sun/ Heat		Cold		Windy	
Rain		Aching		Cloudy	
Other					

PAIN SCALE
NO PAIN ⟶ SEVERE PAIN

0	1	2	3	4	5	6	7	8	9	10

SUSPECTED TRIGGERS

-
-
-
-

-
-
-
-

SYMPTOMS

RELIEF MEASURES

NOTES

CHRONIC PAIN ASSESSMENT

DATE		DAY	
TIME STARTED		TIME ENDED	
TOTAL DURATION			

Mark the location of the pain

LENGTH OF TIME EXPERIENCING THE PAIN?

< 6 Months		6-12 Months	
1-3 Years		3 Years +	

TYPE OF PAIN

Indescribable		Stabbing		Sharp	
Burning		Aching		Prickly	
Numb		Tingling/ Pins & Needles			
Other					

EXTERNAL ENVIROMENTAL FACTORS

Sun/ Heat		Cold		Windy	
Rain		Aching		Cloudy	
Other					

PAIN SCALE
NO PAIN ———————————————————→ SEVERE PAIN

0	1	2	3	4	5	6	7	8	9	10

SUSPECTED TRIGGERS
-
-
-
-

SYMPTOMS

RELIEF MEASURES

NOTES

CHRONIC PAIN ASSESSMENT

DATE		DAY	
TIME STARTED		TIME ENDED	
TOTAL DURATION			

← Mark the location of the pain

LENGTH OF TIME EXPERIENCING THE PAIN?

< 6 Months		6-12 Months	
1-3 Years		3 Years +	

TYPE OF PAIN

Indescribable		Stabbing		Sharp	
Burning		Aching		Prickly	
Numb		Tingling/ Pins & Needles			
Other					

EXTERNAL ENVIROMENTAL FACTORS

Sun/ Heat		Cold		Windy	
Rain		Aching		Cloudy	
Other					

PAIN SCALE
NO PAIN ——————————————————→ SEVERE PAIN

0	1	2	3	4	5	6	7	8	9	10

SUSPECTED TRIGGERS

-
-
-
-

-
-
-
-

SYMPTOMS

RELIEF MEASURES

NOTES

CHRONIC PAIN ASSESSMENT

DATE		DAY	
TIME STARTED		TIME ENDED	
TOTAL DURATION			

Mark the location of the pain

LENGTH OF TIME EXPERIENCING THE PAIN?
< 6 Months		6-12 Months	
1-3 Years		3 Years +	

TYPE OF PAIN
Indescribable		Stabbing		Sharp	
Burning		Aching		Prickly	
Numb		Tingling/ Pins & Needles			
Other					

EXTERNAL ENVIROMENTAL FACTORS
Sun/ Heat		Cold		Windy	
Rain		Aching		Cloudy	
Other					

PAIN SCALE
NO PAIN →→→→→→→→→→→→→→→→→→→→→→→ SEVERE PAIN

0	1	2	3	4	5	6	7	8	9	10

SUSPECTED TRIGGERS
-
-
-
-
-
-
-
-

SYMPTOMS

RELIEF MEASURES

NOTES

CHRONIC PAIN ASSESSMENT

DATE		DAY	
TIME STARTED		TIME ENDED	
TOTAL DURATION			

Mark the location of the pain

LENGTH OF TIME EXPERIENCING THE PAIN?

< 6 Months		6-12 Months	
1-3 Years		3 Years +	

TYPE OF PAIN

Indescribable		Stabbing		Sharp	
Burning		Aching		Prickly	
Numb		Tingling/ Pins & Needles			
Other					

EXTERNAL ENVIROMENTAL FACTORS

Sun/ Heat		Cold		Windy	
Rain		Aching		Cloudy	
Other					

PAIN SCALE
NO PAIN ⟶ SEVERE PAIN

0	1	2	3	4	5	6	7	8	9	10

SUSPECTED TRIGGERS
-
-
-
-

-
-
-
-

SYMPTOMS

RELIEF MEASURES

NOTES

CHRONIC PAIN ASSESSMENT

DATE		DAY	
TIME STARTED		TIME ENDED	
TOTAL DURATION			

Mark the location of the pain

LENGTH OF TIME EXPERIENCING THE PAIN?

< 6 Months		6-12 Months	
1-3 Years		3 Years +	

TYPE OF PAIN

Indescribable	Stabbing		Sharp	
Burning	Aching		Prickly	
Numb	Tingling/ Pins & Needles			
Other				

EXTERNAL ENVIROMENTAL FACTORS

Sun/ Heat		Cold		Windy	
Rain		Aching		Cloudy	
Other					

PAIN SCALE

NO PAIN ──────────────────────→ SEVERE PAIN

0	1	2	3	4	5	6	7	8	9	10

SUSPECTED TRIGGERS

-
-
-
-

SYMPTOMS

RELIEF MEASURES

NOTES

CHRONIC PAIN ASSESSMENT

DATE		DAY	
TIME STARTED		TIME ENDED	
TOTAL DURATION			

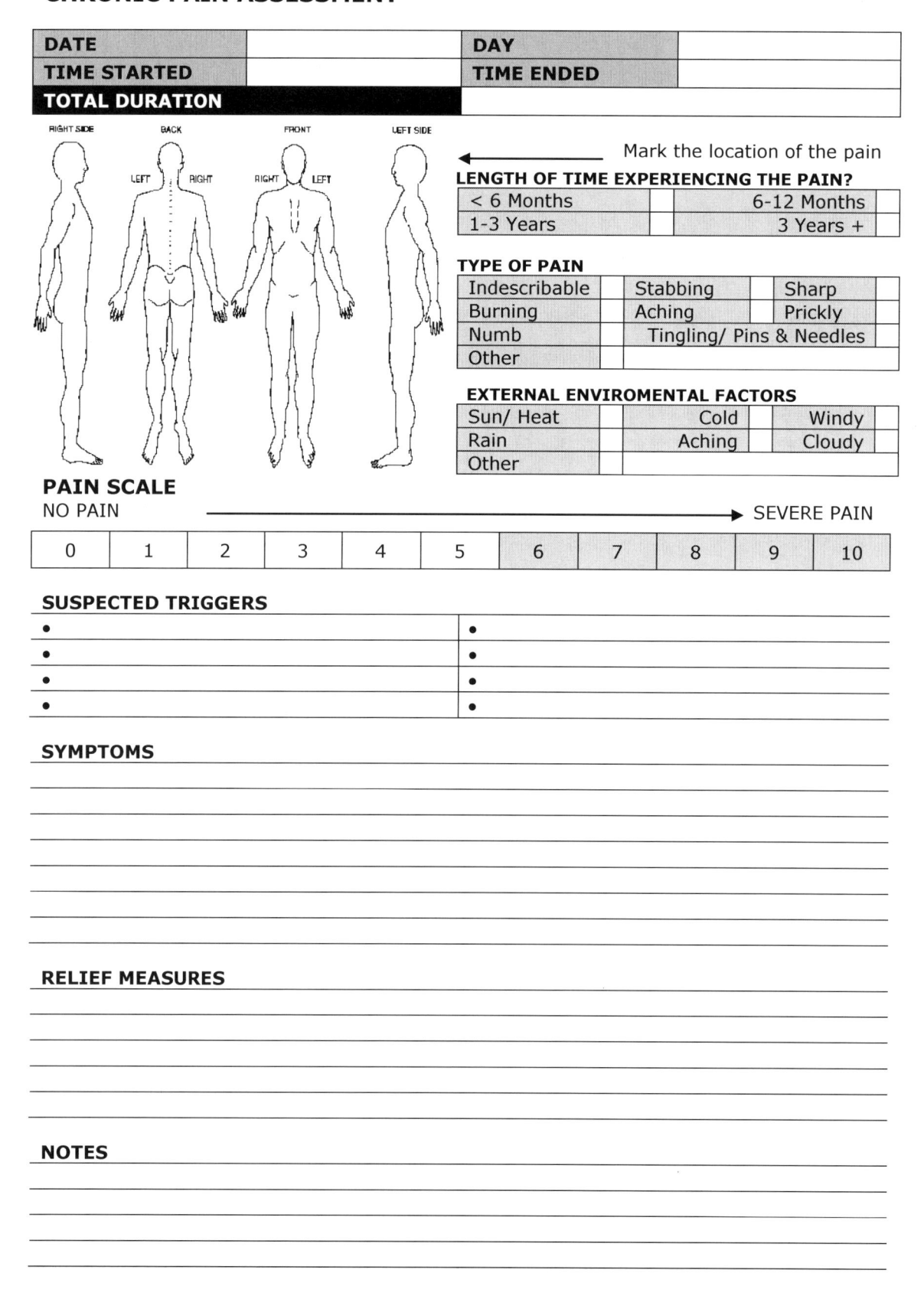

Mark the location of the pain

LENGTH OF TIME EXPERIENCING THE PAIN?

< 6 Months		6-12 Months	
1-3 Years		3 Years +	

TYPE OF PAIN

Indescribable		Stabbing		Sharp	
Burning		Aching		Prickly	
Numb		Tingling/ Pins & Needles			
Other					

EXTERNAL ENVIROMENTAL FACTORS

Sun/ Heat		Cold		Windy	
Rain		Aching		Cloudy	
Other					

PAIN SCALE

NO PAIN ⟶ SEVERE PAIN

0	1	2	3	4	5	6	7	8	9	10

SUSPECTED TRIGGERS

-
-
-
-

-
-
-
-

SYMPTOMS

RELIEF MEASURES

NOTES

CHRONIC PAIN ASSESSMENT

DATE		DAY	
TIME STARTED		TIME ENDED	
TOTAL DURATION			

Mark the location of the pain

LENGTH OF TIME EXPERIENCING THE PAIN?
< 6 Months		6-12 Months	
1-3 Years		3 Years +	

TYPE OF PAIN
Indescribable		Stabbing		Sharp	
Burning		Aching		Prickly	
Numb		Tingling/ Pins & Needles			
Other					

EXTERNAL ENVIROMENTAL FACTORS
Sun/ Heat		Cold		Windy	
Rain		Aching		Cloudy	
Other					

PAIN SCALE
NO PAIN ⟶ SEVERE PAIN

0	1	2	3	4	5	6	7	8	9	10

SUSPECTED TRIGGERS
-
-
-
-

SYMPTOMS

RELIEF MEASURES

NOTES

CHRONIC PAIN ASSESSMENT

DATE		DAY	
TIME STARTED		TIME ENDED	
TOTAL DURATION			

Mark the location of the pain

LENGTH OF TIME EXPERIENCING THE PAIN?
< 6 Months		6-12 Months	
1-3 Years		3 Years +	

TYPE OF PAIN
Indescribable		Stabbing		Sharp	
Burning		Aching		Prickly	
Numb		Tingling/ Pins & Needles			
Other					

EXTERNAL ENVIROMENTAL FACTORS
Sun/ Heat		Cold		Windy	
Rain		Aching		Cloudy	
Other					

PAIN SCALE
NO PAIN ⟶ SEVERE PAIN

0	1	2	3	4	5	6	7	8	9	10

SUSPECTED TRIGGERS
-
-
-
-

-
-
-
-

SYMPTOMS

RELIEF MEASURES

NOTES

CHRONIC PAIN ASSESSMENT

DATE		DAY	
TIME STARTED		TIME ENDED	
TOTAL DURATION			

Mark the location of the pain

LENGTH OF TIME EXPERIENCING THE PAIN?

< 6 Months		6-12 Months	
1-3 Years		3 Years +	

TYPE OF PAIN

Indescribable		Stabbing		Sharp	
Burning		Aching		Prickly	
Numb		Tingling/ Pins & Needles			
Other					

EXTERNAL ENVIROMENTAL FACTORS

Sun/ Heat		Cold		Windy	
Rain		Aching		Cloudy	
Other					

PAIN SCALE

NO PAIN ⟶ SEVERE PAIN

0	1	2	3	4	5	6	7	8	9	10

SUSPECTED TRIGGERS

-
-
-
-

-
-
-
-

SYMPTOMS

RELIEF MEASURES

NOTES

CHRONIC PAIN ASSESSMENT

DATE		DAY	
TIME STARTED		TIME ENDED	
TOTAL DURATION			

Mark the location of the pain

RIGHT SIDE BACK FRONT LEFT SIDE
LEFT RIGHT RIGHT LEFT

LENGTH OF TIME EXPERIENCING THE PAIN?

< 6 Months		6-12 Months	
1-3 Years		3 Years +	

TYPE OF PAIN

Indescribable		Stabbing		Sharp	
Burning		Aching		Prickly	
Numb		Tingling/ Pins & Needles			
Other					

EXTERNAL ENVIROMENTAL FACTORS

Sun/ Heat		Cold		Windy	
Rain		Aching		Cloudy	
Other					

PAIN SCALE
NO PAIN ⟶ SEVERE PAIN

0	1	2	3	4	5	6	7	8	9	10

SUSPECTED TRIGGERS

-
-
-
-

-
-
-
-

SYMPTOMS

RELIEF MEASURES

NOTES

CHRONIC PAIN ASSESSMENT

DATE		DAY	
TIME STARTED		**TIME ENDED**	
TOTAL DURATION			

RIGHT SIDE BACK FRONT LEFT SIDE

← Mark the location of the pain

LENGTH OF TIME EXPERIENCING THE PAIN?

< 6 Months		6-12 Months	
1-3 Years		3 Years +	

TYPE OF PAIN

Indescribable		Stabbing		Sharp	
Burning		Aching		Prickly	
Numb		Tingling/ Pins & Needles			
Other					

EXTERNAL ENVIRONMENTAL FACTORS

Sun/ Heat		Cold		Windy	
Rain		Aching		Cloudy	
Other					

PAIN SCALE

NO PAIN ──────────────→ SEVERE PAIN

0	1	2	3	4	5	6	7	8	9	10

SUSPECTED TRIGGERS

-
-
-
-

-
-
-
-

SYMPTOMS

RELIEF MEASURES

NOTES

CHRONIC PAIN ASSESSMENT

DATE		DAY	
TIME STARTED		TIME ENDED	
TOTAL DURATION			

← Mark the location of the pain

LENGTH OF TIME EXPERIENCING THE PAIN?

< 6 Months		6-12 Months	
1-3 Years		3 Years +	

TYPE OF PAIN

Indescribable		Stabbing		Sharp	
Burning		Aching		Prickly	
Numb		Tingling/ Pins & Needles			
Other					

EXTERNAL ENVIROMENTAL FACTORS

Sun/ Heat		Cold		Windy	
Rain		Aching		Cloudy	
Other					

PAIN SCALE
NO PAIN ⟶ SEVERE PAIN

0	1	2	3	4	5	6	7	8	9	10

SUSPECTED TRIGGERS

-
-
-
-

-
-
-
-

SYMPTOMS

RELIEF MEASURES

NOTES

CHRONIC PAIN ASSESSMENT

DATE		DAY	
TIME STARTED		TIME ENDED	
TOTAL DURATION			

Mark the location of the pain

LENGTH OF TIME EXPERIENCING THE PAIN?

< 6 Months		6-12 Months	
1-3 Years		3 Years +	

TYPE OF PAIN

Indescribable		Stabbing		Sharp	
Burning		Aching		Prickly	
Numb		Tingling/ Pins & Needles			
Other					

EXTERNAL ENVIROMENTAL FACTORS

Sun/ Heat		Cold		Windy	
Rain		Aching		Cloudy	
Other					

PAIN SCALE
NO PAIN ⟶ SEVERE PAIN

0	1	2	3	4	5	6	7	8	9	10

SUSPECTED TRIGGERS
-
-
-
-

SYMPTOMS

RELIEF MEASURES

NOTES

CHRONIC PAIN ASSESSMENT

DATE		DAY	
TIME STARTED		TIME ENDED	
TOTAL DURATION			

Mark the location of the pain

LENGTH OF TIME EXPERIENCING THE PAIN?

< 6 Months		6-12 Months	
1-3 Years		3 Years +	

TYPE OF PAIN

Indescribable		Stabbing		Sharp	
Burning		Aching		Prickly	
Numb		Tingling/ Pins & Needles			
Other					

EXTERNAL ENVIROMENTAL FACTORS

Sun/ Heat		Cold		Windy	
Rain		Aching		Cloudy	
Other					

PAIN SCALE
NO PAIN ⟶ SEVERE PAIN

0	1	2	3	4	5	6	7	8	9	10

SUSPECTED TRIGGERS

-
-
-
-

-
-
-
-

SYMPTOMS

RELIEF MEASURES

NOTES

Page 35

CHRONIC PAIN ASSESSMENT

DATE		DAY	
TIME STARTED		TIME ENDED	
TOTAL DURATION			

RIGHT SIDE BACK FRONT LEFT SIDE

← Mark the location of the pain

LENGTH OF TIME EXPERIENCING THE PAIN?

< 6 Months		6-12 Months	
1-3 Years		3 Years +	

TYPE OF PAIN

Indescribable		Stabbing		Sharp	
Burning		Aching		Prickly	
Numb		Tingling/ Pins & Needles			
Other					

EXTERNAL ENVIROMENTAL FACTORS

Sun/ Heat		Cold		Windy	
Rain		Aching		Cloudy	
Other					

PAIN SCALE

NO PAIN ──────────────────→ SEVERE PAIN

0	1	2	3	4	5	6	7	8	9	10

SUSPECTED TRIGGERS

-
-
-
-
-
-
-
-

SYMPTOMS

RELIEF MEASURES

NOTES

CHRONIC PAIN ASSESSMENT

DATE		DAY	
TIME STARTED		TIME ENDED	
TOTAL DURATION			

Mark the location of the pain

LENGTH OF TIME EXPERIENCING THE PAIN?
< 6 Months		6-12 Months	
1-3 Years		3 Years +	

TYPE OF PAIN
Indescribable		Stabbing		Sharp	
Burning		Aching		Prickly	
Numb		Tingling/ Pins & Needles			
Other					

EXTERNAL ENVIROMENTAL FACTORS
Sun/ Heat		Cold		Windy	
Rain		Aching		Cloudy	
Other					

PAIN SCALE
NO PAIN ──────────────────────────→ SEVERE PAIN

0	1	2	3	4	5	6	7	8	9	10

SUSPECTED TRIGGERS
-
-
-
-

-
-
-
-

SYMPTOMS

RELIEF MEASURES

NOTES

CHRONIC PAIN ASSESSMENT

DATE		DAY	
TIME STARTED		**TIME ENDED**	
TOTAL DURATION			

RIGHT SIDE BACK FRONT LEFT SIDE

⬅ Mark the location of the pain

LENGTH OF TIME EXPERIENCING THE PAIN?

< 6 Months		6-12 Months	
1-3 Years		3 Years +	

TYPE OF PAIN

Indescribable		Stabbing		Sharp	
Burning		Aching		Prickly	
Numb		Tingling/ Pins & Needles			
Other					

EXTERNAL ENVIROMENTAL FACTORS

Sun/ Heat		Cold		Windy	
Rain		Aching		Cloudy	
Other					

PAIN SCALE

NO PAIN ⟶ SEVERE PAIN

0	1	2	3	4	5	6	7	8	9	10

SUSPECTED TRIGGERS

-
-
-
-

-
-
-
-

SYMPTOMS

RELIEF MEASURES

NOTES

CHRONIC PAIN ASSESSMENT

DATE		DAY	
TIME STARTED		TIME ENDED	
TOTAL DURATION			

Mark the location of the pain

LENGTH OF TIME EXPERIENCING THE PAIN?

< 6 Months		6-12 Months	
1-3 Years		3 Years +	

TYPE OF PAIN

Indescribable		Stabbing		Sharp	
Burning		Aching		Prickly	
Numb		Tingling/ Pins & Needles			
Other					

EXTERNAL ENVIROMENTAL FACTORS

Sun/ Heat		Cold		Windy	
Rain		Aching		Cloudy	
Other					

PAIN SCALE
NO PAIN → SEVERE PAIN

0	1	2	3	4	5	6	7	8	9	10

SUSPECTED TRIGGERS
-
-
-
-

-
-
-
-

SYMPTOMS

RELIEF MEASURES

NOTES

CHRONIC PAIN ASSESSMENT

DATE		DAY	
TIME STARTED		TIME ENDED	
TOTAL DURATION			

Mark the location of the pain

LENGTH OF TIME EXPERIENCING THE PAIN?

< 6 Months		6-12 Months	
1-3 Years		3 Years +	

TYPE OF PAIN

Indescribable		Stabbing		Sharp	
Burning		Aching		Prickly	
Numb		Tingling/ Pins & Needles			
Other					

EXTERNAL ENVIROMENTAL FACTORS

Sun/ Heat		Cold		Windy	
Rain		Aching		Cloudy	
Other					

PAIN SCALE
NO PAIN ⟶ SEVERE PAIN

0	1	2	3	4	5	6	7	8	9	10

SUSPECTED TRIGGERS
-
-
-
-
-
-
-
-

SYMPTOMS

RELIEF MEASURES

NOTES

CHRONIC PAIN ASSESSMENT

DATE		DAY	
TIME STARTED		TIME ENDED	
TOTAL DURATION			

Mark the location of the pain

LENGTH OF TIME EXPERIENCING THE PAIN?

< 6 Months		6-12 Months	
1-3 Years		3 Years +	

TYPE OF PAIN

Indescribable		Stabbing		Sharp	
Burning		Aching		Prickly	
Numb		Tingling/ Pins & Needles			
Other					

EXTERNAL ENVIROMENTAL FACTORS

Sun/ Heat		Cold		Windy	
Rain		Aching		Cloudy	
Other					

PAIN SCALE
NO PAIN ⟶ SEVERE PAIN

0	1	2	3	4	5	6	7	8	9	10

SUSPECTED TRIGGERS
-
-
-
-

SYMPTOMS

RELIEF MEASURES

NOTES

CHRONIC PAIN ASSESSMENT

DATE		DAY	
TIME STARTED		TIME ENDED	
TOTAL DURATION			

RIGHT SIDE BACK FRONT LEFT SIDE

⬅ Mark the location of the pain

LENGTH OF TIME EXPERIENCING THE PAIN?

< 6 Months		6-12 Months	
1-3 Years		3 Years +	

TYPE OF PAIN

Indescribable	Stabbing	Sharp
Burning	Aching	Prickly
Numb	Tingling/ Pins & Needles	
Other		

EXTERNAL ENVIROMENTAL FACTORS

Sun/ Heat	Cold	Windy
Rain	Aching	Cloudy
Other		

PAIN SCALE
NO PAIN ⟶ SEVERE PAIN

0	1	2	3	4	5	6	7	8	9	10

SUSPECTED TRIGGERS
-
-
-
-
-
-
-
-

SYMPTOMS

RELIEF MEASURES

NOTES

CHRONIC PAIN ASSESSMENT

DATE		DAY	
TIME STARTED		TIME ENDED	
TOTAL DURATION			

← Mark the location of the pain

LENGTH OF TIME EXPERIENCING THE PAIN?

< 6 Months		6-12 Months	
1-3 Years		3 Years +	

TYPE OF PAIN

Indescribable		Stabbing		Sharp	
Burning		Aching		Prickly	
Numb		Tingling/ Pins & Needles			
Other					

EXTERNAL ENVIROMENTAL FACTORS

Sun/ Heat		Cold		Windy	
Rain		Aching		Cloudy	
Other					

PAIN SCALE
NO PAIN ⟶ SEVERE PAIN

0	1	2	3	4	5	6	7	8	9	10

SUSPECTED TRIGGERS
-
-
-
-

-
-
-
-

SYMPTOMS

RELIEF MEASURES

NOTES

CHRONIC PAIN ASSESSMENT

DATE		DAY	
TIME STARTED		TIME ENDED	
TOTAL DURATION			

Mark the location of the pain

LENGTH OF TIME EXPERIENCING THE PAIN?
< 6 Months		6-12 Months	
1-3 Years		3 Years +	

TYPE OF PAIN
Indescribable		Stabbing		Sharp	
Burning		Aching		Prickly	
Numb		Tingling/ Pins & Needles			
Other					

EXTERNAL ENVIROMENTAL FACTORS
Sun/ Heat		Cold		Windy	
Rain		Aching		Cloudy	
Other					

PAIN SCALE
NO PAIN ⟶ SEVERE PAIN

0	1	2	3	4	5	6	7	8	9	10

SUSPECTED TRIGGERS
-
-
-
-
-
-
-
-

SYMPTOMS

RELIEF MEASURES

NOTES

CHRONIC PAIN ASSESSMENT

DATE		DAY	
TIME STARTED		TIME ENDED	
TOTAL DURATION			

Mark the location of the pain

LENGTH OF TIME EXPERIENCING THE PAIN?

< 6 Months		6-12 Months	
1-3 Years		3 Years +	

TYPE OF PAIN

Indescribable		Stabbing		Sharp	
Burning		Aching		Prickly	
Numb		Tingling/ Pins & Needles			
Other					

EXTERNAL ENVIROMENTAL FACTORS

Sun/ Heat		Cold		Windy	
Rain		Aching		Cloudy	
Other					

PAIN SCALE
NO PAIN ⟶ SEVERE PAIN

0	1	2	3	4	5	6	7	8	9	10

SUSPECTED TRIGGERS
-
-
-
-
-
-
-
-

SYMPTOMS

RELIEF MEASURES

NOTES

CHRONIC PAIN ASSESSMENT

DATE		DAY	
TIME STARTED		**TIME ENDED**	
TOTAL DURATION			

RIGHT SIDE   BACK   FRONT   LEFT SIDE

⬅ Mark the location of the pain

LENGTH OF TIME EXPERIENCING THE PAIN?

< 6 Months		6-12 Months	
1-3 Years		3 Years +	

TYPE OF PAIN

Indescribable		Stabbing		Sharp	
Burning		Aching		Prickly	
Numb		Tingling/ Pins & Needles			
Other					

EXTERNAL ENVIROMENTAL FACTORS

Sun/ Heat		Cold		Windy	
Rain		Aching		Cloudy	
Other					

PAIN SCALE

NO PAIN ⟶ SEVERE PAIN

0	1	2	3	4	5	6	7	8	9	10

SUSPECTED TRIGGERS

-
-
-
-

-
-
-
-

SYMPTOMS

RELIEF MEASURES

NOTES

CHRONIC PAIN ASSESSMENT

DATE		DAY	
TIME STARTED		TIME ENDED	
TOTAL DURATION			

Mark the location of the pain

LENGTH OF TIME EXPERIENCING THE PAIN?

< 6 Months		6-12 Months	
1-3 Years		3 Years +	

TYPE OF PAIN

Indescribable		Stabbing		Sharp	
Burning		Aching		Prickly	
Numb		Tingling/ Pins & Needles			
Other					

EXTERNAL ENVIROMENTAL FACTORS

Sun/ Heat		Cold		Windy	
Rain		Aching		Cloudy	
Other					

PAIN SCALE
NO PAIN ⟶ SEVERE PAIN

0	1	2	3	4	5	6	7	8	9	10

SUSPECTED TRIGGERS

-
-
-
-

-
-
-
-

SYMPTOMS

RELIEF MEASURES

NOTES

CHRONIC PAIN ASSESSMENT

DATE		DAY	
TIME STARTED		TIME ENDED	
TOTAL DURATION			

Mark the location of the pain

LENGTH OF TIME EXPERIENCING THE PAIN?

< 6 Months		6-12 Months	
1-3 Years		3 Years +	

TYPE OF PAIN

Indescribable		Stabbing		Sharp	
Burning		Aching		Prickly	
Numb		Tingling/ Pins & Needles			
Other					

EXTERNAL ENVIROMENTAL FACTORS

Sun/ Heat		Cold		Windy	
Rain		Aching		Cloudy	
Other					

PAIN SCALE

NO PAIN ──────────────────→ SEVERE PAIN

0	1	2	3	4	5	6	7	8	9	10

SUSPECTED TRIGGERS

-
-
-
-

SYMPTOMS

RELIEF MEASURES

NOTES

CHRONIC PAIN ASSESSMENT

DATE		DAY	
TIME STARTED		TIME ENDED	
TOTAL DURATION			

Mark the location of the pain

LENGTH OF TIME EXPERIENCING THE PAIN?

< 6 Months		6-12 Months	
1-3 Years		3 Years +	

TYPE OF PAIN

Indescribable		Stabbing		Sharp	
Burning		Aching		Prickly	
Numb		Tingling/ Pins & Needles			
Other					

EXTERNAL ENVIROMENTAL FACTORS

Sun/ Heat		Cold		Windy	
Rain		Aching		Cloudy	
Other					

PAIN SCALE
NO PAIN ──────────────────────────→ SEVERE PAIN

0	1	2	3	4	5	6	7	8	9	10

SUSPECTED TRIGGERS

-
-
-
-

-
-
-
-

SYMPTOMS

RELIEF MEASURES

NOTES

CHRONIC PAIN ASSESSMENT

DATE		DAY	
TIME STARTED		**TIME ENDED**	
TOTAL DURATION			

← Mark the location of the pain

LENGTH OF TIME EXPERIENCING THE PAIN?

< 6 Months		6-12 Months	
1-3 Years		3 Years +	

TYPE OF PAIN

Indescribable		Stabbing		Sharp	
Burning		Aching		Prickly	
Numb		Tingling/ Pins & Needles			
Other					

EXTERNAL ENVIROMENTAL FACTORS

Sun/ Heat		Cold		Windy	
Rain		Aching		Cloudy	
Other					

PAIN SCALE

NO PAIN ⟶ SEVERE PAIN

0	1	2	3	4	5	6	7	8	9	10

SUSPECTED TRIGGERS

-
-
-
-

-
-
-
-

SYMPTOMS

RELIEF MEASURES

NOTES

CHRONIC PAIN ASSESSMENT

DATE		DAY	
TIME STARTED		TIME ENDED	
TOTAL DURATION			

Mark the location of the pain

LENGTH OF TIME EXPERIENCING THE PAIN?

< 6 Months		6-12 Months	
1-3 Years		3 Years +	

TYPE OF PAIN

Indescribable		Stabbing		Sharp	
Burning		Aching		Prickly	
Numb		Tingling/ Pins & Needles			
Other					

EXTERNAL ENVIROMENTAL FACTORS

Sun/ Heat		Cold		Windy	
Rain		Aching		Cloudy	
Other					

PAIN SCALE
NO PAIN → SEVERE PAIN

0	1	2	3	4	5	6	7	8	9	10

SUSPECTED TRIGGERS

-
-
-
-

-
-
-
-

SYMPTOMS

_____
_____
_____
_____
_____
_____
_____
_____

RELIEF MEASURES

_____
_____
_____
_____
_____
_____

NOTES

_____
_____
_____
_____
_____

CHRONIC PAIN ASSESSMENT

DATE		DAY	
TIME STARTED		TIME ENDED	
TOTAL DURATION			

← Mark the location of the pain

LENGTH OF TIME EXPERIENCING THE PAIN?

< 6 Months		6-12 Months	
1-3 Years		3 Years +	

TYPE OF PAIN

Indescribable		Stabbing		Sharp	
Burning		Aching		Prickly	
Numb		Tingling/ Pins & Needles			
Other					

EXTERNAL ENVIRONMENTAL FACTORS

Sun/ Heat		Cold		Windy	
Rain		Aching		Cloudy	
Other					

PAIN SCALE

NO PAIN ⟶ SEVERE PAIN

0	1	2	3	4	5	6	7	8	9	10

SUSPECTED TRIGGERS

-
-
-
-

-
-
-
-

SYMPTOMS

RELIEF MEASURES

NOTES

CHRONIC PAIN ASSESSMENT

DATE		DAY	
TIME STARTED		TIME ENDED	
TOTAL DURATION			

Mark the location of the pain

LENGTH OF TIME EXPERIENCING THE PAIN?

< 6 Months		6-12 Months	
1-3 Years		3 Years +	

TYPE OF PAIN

Indescribable		Stabbing		Sharp	
Burning		Aching		Prickly	
Numb		Tingling/ Pins & Needles			
Other					

EXTERNAL ENVIROMENTAL FACTORS

Sun/ Heat		Cold		Windy	
Rain		Aching		Cloudy	
Other					

PAIN SCALE
NO PAIN ⟶ SEVERE PAIN

0	1	2	3	4	5	6	7	8	9	10

SUSPECTED TRIGGERS
-
-
-
-

-
-
-
-

SYMPTOMS

RELIEF MEASURES

NOTES

CHRONIC PAIN ASSESSMENT

DATE		DAY	
TIME STARTED		**TIME ENDED**	
TOTAL DURATION			

← Mark the location of the pain

LENGTH OF TIME EXPERIENCING THE PAIN?

< 6 Months		6-12 Months	
1-3 Years		3 Years +	

TYPE OF PAIN

Indescribable		Stabbing		Sharp	
Burning		Aching		Prickly	
Numb		Tingling/ Pins & Needles			
Other					

EXTERNAL ENVIRONMENTAL FACTORS

Sun/ Heat		Cold		Windy	
Rain		Aching		Cloudy	
Other					

PAIN SCALE

NO PAIN ──────────────────→ SEVERE PAIN

0	1	2	3	4	5	6	7	8	9	10

SUSPECTED TRIGGERS
-
-
-
-
-
-
-
-

SYMPTOMS

RELIEF MEASURES

NOTES

CHRONIC PAIN ASSESSMENT

DATE		DAY	
TIME STARTED		**TIME ENDED**	
TOTAL DURATION			

Mark the location of the pain

LENGTH OF TIME EXPERIENCING THE PAIN?

< 6 Months		6-12 Months	
1-3 Years		3 Years +	

TYPE OF PAIN

Indescribable		Stabbing		Sharp	
Burning		Aching		Prickly	
Numb		Tingling/ Pins & Needles			
Other					

EXTERNAL ENVIROMENTAL FACTORS

Sun/ Heat		Cold		Windy	
Rain		Aching		Cloudy	
Other					

PAIN SCALE
NO PAIN ⟶ SEVERE PAIN

0	1	2	3	4	5	6	7	8	9	10

SUSPECTED TRIGGERS

-
-
-
-

-
-
-
-

SYMPTOMS

RELIEF MEASURES

NOTES

CHRONIC PAIN ASSESSMENT

DATE		DAY	
TIME STARTED		TIME ENDED	
TOTAL DURATION			

Mark the location of the pain

LENGTH OF TIME EXPERIENCING THE PAIN?

< 6 Months		6-12 Months	
1-3 Years		3 Years +	

TYPE OF PAIN

Indescribable		Stabbing		Sharp	
Burning		Aching		Prickly	
Numb		Tingling/ Pins & Needles			
Other					

EXTERNAL ENVIROMENTAL FACTORS

Sun/ Heat		Cold		Windy	
Rain		Aching		Cloudy	
Other					

PAIN SCALE
NO PAIN ⟶ SEVERE PAIN

0	1	2	3	4	5	6	7	8	9	10

SUSPECTED TRIGGERS
-
-
-
-
-
-
-
-

SYMPTOMS

RELIEF MEASURES

NOTES

CHRONIC PAIN ASSESSMENT

DATE		DAY	
TIME STARTED		TIME ENDED	
TOTAL DURATION			

← Mark the location of the pain

LENGTH OF TIME EXPERIENCING THE PAIN?
< 6 Months		6-12 Months	
1-3 Years		3 Years +	

TYPE OF PAIN
Indescribable		Stabbing		Sharp	
Burning		Aching		Prickly	
Numb		Tingling/ Pins & Needles			
Other					

EXTERNAL ENVIROMENTAL FACTORS
Sun/ Heat		Cold		Windy	
Rain		Aching		Cloudy	
Other					

PAIN SCALE
NO PAIN ⟶ SEVERE PAIN

0	1	2	3	4	5	6	7	8	9	10

SUSPECTED TRIGGERS
-
-
-
-

SYMPTOMS

RELIEF MEASURES

NOTES

CHRONIC PAIN ASSESSMENT

DATE		DAY	
TIME STARTED		TIME ENDED	
TOTAL DURATION			

Mark the location of the pain

LENGTH OF TIME EXPERIENCING THE PAIN?

< 6 Months		6-12 Months	
1-3 Years		3 Years +	

TYPE OF PAIN

Indescribable		Stabbing		Sharp	
Burning		Aching		Prickly	
Numb		Tingling/ Pins & Needles			
Other					

EXTERNAL ENVIROMENTAL FACTORS

Sun/ Heat		Cold		Windy	
Rain		Aching		Cloudy	
Other					

PAIN SCALE
NO PAIN ──────────────────────────────→ SEVERE PAIN

0	1	2	3	4	5	6	7	8	9	10

SUSPECTED TRIGGERS
-
-
-
-

SYMPTOMS

RELIEF MEASURES

NOTES

CHRONIC PAIN ASSESSMENT

DATE		DAY	
TIME STARTED		TIME ENDED	
TOTAL DURATION			

Mark the location of the pain

LENGTH OF TIME EXPERIENCING THE PAIN?

< 6 Months		6-12 Months	
1-3 Years		3 Years +	

TYPE OF PAIN

Indescribable		Stabbing		Sharp	
Burning		Aching		Prickly	
Numb		Tingling/ Pins & Needles			
Other					

EXTERNAL ENVIROMENTAL FACTORS

Sun/ Heat		Cold		Windy	
Rain		Aching		Cloudy	
Other					

PAIN SCALE
NO PAIN → SEVERE PAIN

0	1	2	3	4	5	6	7	8	9	10

SUSPECTED TRIGGERS
-
-
-
-

SYMPTOMS

RELIEF MEASURES

NOTES

CHRONIC PAIN ASSESSMENT

DATE		DAY	
TIME STARTED		TIME ENDED	
TOTAL DURATION			

Mark the location of the pain

LENGTH OF TIME EXPERIENCING THE PAIN?

< 6 Months		6-12 Months	
1-3 Years		3 Years +	

TYPE OF PAIN

Indescribable		Stabbing		Sharp	
Burning		Aching		Prickly	
Numb		Tingling/ Pins & Needles			
Other					

EXTERNAL ENVIROMENTAL FACTORS

Sun/ Heat		Cold		Windy	
Rain		Aching		Cloudy	
Other					

PAIN SCALE

NO PAIN ⟶ SEVERE PAIN

0	1	2	3	4	5	6	7	8	9	10

SUSPECTED TRIGGERS

-
-
-
-

SYMPTOMS

RELIEF MEASURES

NOTES

CHRONIC PAIN ASSESSMENT

DATE		DAY	
TIME STARTED		TIME ENDED	
TOTAL DURATION			

← Mark the location of the pain

LENGTH OF TIME EXPERIENCING THE PAIN?

< 6 Months		6-12 Months	
1-3 Years		3 Years +	

TYPE OF PAIN

Indescribable		Stabbing		Sharp	
Burning		Aching		Prickly	
Numb		Tingling/ Pins & Needles			
Other					

EXTERNAL ENVIROMENTAL FACTORS

Sun/ Heat		Cold		Windy	
Rain		Aching		Cloudy	
Other					

PAIN SCALE
NO PAIN ⟶ SEVERE PAIN

0	1	2	3	4	5	6	7	8	9	10

SUSPECTED TRIGGERS
-
-
-
-
-
-
-
-

SYMPTOMS

RELIEF MEASURES

NOTES

CHRONIC PAIN ASSESSMENT

DATE		DAY	
TIME STARTED		**TIME ENDED**	
TOTAL DURATION			

RIGHT SIDE BACK FRONT LEFT SIDE

⬅ Mark the location of the pain

LENGTH OF TIME EXPERIENCING THE PAIN?

< 6 Months		6-12 Months	
1-3 Years		3 Years +	

TYPE OF PAIN

Indescribable		Stabbing		Sharp	
Burning		Aching		Prickly	
Numb		Tingling/ Pins & Needles			
Other					

EXTERNAL ENVIROMENTAL FACTORS

Sun/ Heat		Cold		Windy	
Rain		Aching		Cloudy	
Other					

PAIN SCALE
NO PAIN ⟶ SEVERE PAIN

0	1	2	3	4	5	6	7	8	9	10

SUSPECTED TRIGGERS
-
-
-
-
-
-
-
-

SYMPTOMS

RELIEF MEASURES

NOTES

CHRONIC PAIN ASSESSMENT

DATE		DAY	
TIME STARTED		TIME ENDED	
TOTAL DURATION			

Mark the location of the pain

LENGTH OF TIME EXPERIENCING THE PAIN?

< 6 Months		6-12 Months	
1-3 Years		3 Years +	

TYPE OF PAIN

Indescribable		Stabbing		Sharp	
Burning		Aching		Prickly	
Numb		Tingling/ Pins & Needles			
Other					

EXTERNAL ENVIROMENTAL FACTORS

Sun/ Heat		Cold		Windy	
Rain		Aching		Cloudy	
Other					

PAIN SCALE
NO PAIN ──────────────────────────► SEVERE PAIN

0	1	2	3	4	5	6	7	8	9	10

SUSPECTED TRIGGERS
-
-
-
-

-
-
-
-

SYMPTOMS
_____
_____
_____
_____
_____
_____
_____

RELIEF MEASURES
_____
_____
_____
_____
_____
_____

NOTES
_____
_____
_____
_____
_____

CHRONIC PAIN ASSESSMENT

DATE		DAY	
TIME STARTED		**TIME ENDED**	
TOTAL DURATION			

← Mark the location of the pain

LENGTH OF TIME EXPERIENCING THE PAIN?

< 6 Months		6-12 Months	
1-3 Years		3 Years +	

TYPE OF PAIN

Indescribable		Stabbing		Sharp	
Burning		Aching		Prickly	
Numb		Tingling/ Pins & Needles			
Other					

EXTERNAL ENVIROMENTAL FACTORS

Sun/ Heat		Cold		Windy	
Rain		Aching		Cloudy	
Other					

PAIN SCALE
NO PAIN ⟶ SEVERE PAIN

0	1	2	3	4	5	6	7	8	9	10

SUSPECTED TRIGGERS

-
-
-
-

SYMPTOMS

RELIEF MEASURES

NOTES

Page 64

CHRONIC PAIN ASSESSMENT

DATE		DAY	
TIME STARTED		TIME ENDED	
TOTAL DURATION			

RIGHT SIDE　BACK　FRONT　LEFT SIDE
LEFT　RIGHT　RIGHT　LEFT

← Mark the location of the pain

LENGTH OF TIME EXPERIENCING THE PAIN?

< 6 Months		6-12 Months	
1-3 Years		3 Years +	

TYPE OF PAIN

Indescribable		Stabbing		Sharp	
Burning		Aching		Prickly	
Numb		Tingling/ Pins & Needles			
Other					

EXTERNAL ENVIROMENTAL FACTORS

Sun/ Heat		Cold		Windy	
Rain		Aching		Cloudy	
Other					

PAIN SCALE
NO PAIN ⟶ SEVERE PAIN

0	1	2	3	4	5	6	7	8	9	10

SUSPECTED TRIGGERS
-
-
-
-

-
-
-
-

SYMPTOMS

RELIEF MEASURES

NOTES

CHRONIC PAIN ASSESSMENT

DATE		DAY	
TIME STARTED		**TIME ENDED**	
TOTAL DURATION			

Mark the location of the pain

LENGTH OF TIME EXPERIENCING THE PAIN?

< 6 Months		6-12 Months	
1-3 Years		3 Years +	

TYPE OF PAIN

Indescribable		Stabbing		Sharp	
Burning		Aching		Prickly	
Numb		Tingling/ Pins & Needles			
Other					

EXTERNAL ENVIROMENTAL FACTORS

Sun/ Heat		Cold		Windy	
Rain		Aching		Cloudy	
Other					

PAIN SCALE
NO PAIN ⟶ SEVERE PAIN

0	1	2	3	4	5	6	7	8	9	10

SUSPECTED TRIGGERS
-
-
-
-

-
-
-
-

SYMPTOMS

RELIEF MEASURES

NOTES

CHRONIC PAIN ASSESSMENT

DATE		DAY	
TIME STARTED		**TIME ENDED**	
TOTAL DURATION			

Mark the location of the pain

LENGTH OF TIME EXPERIENCING THE PAIN?

< 6 Months		6-12 Months	
1-3 Years		3 Years +	

TYPE OF PAIN

Indescribable		Stabbing		Sharp	
Burning		Aching		Prickly	
Numb		Tingling/ Pins & Needles			
Other					

EXTERNAL ENVIROMENTAL FACTORS

Sun/ Heat		Cold		Windy	
Rain		Aching		Cloudy	
Other					

PAIN SCALE
NO PAIN → SEVERE PAIN

0	1	2	3	4	5	6	7	8	9	10

SUSPECTED TRIGGERS

-
-
-
-

SYMPTOMS

RELIEF MEASURES

NOTES

CHRONIC PAIN ASSESSMENT

DATE		DAY	
TIME STARTED		TIME ENDED	
TOTAL DURATION			

Mark the location of the pain

LENGTH OF TIME EXPERIENCING THE PAIN?

< 6 Months		6-12 Months	
1-3 Years		3 Years +	

TYPE OF PAIN

Indescribable		Stabbing		Sharp	
Burning		Aching		Prickly	
Numb		Tingling/ Pins & Needles			
Other					

EXTERNAL ENVIROMENTAL FACTORS

Sun/ Heat		Cold		Windy	
Rain		Aching		Cloudy	
Other					

PAIN SCALE
NO PAIN ⟶ SEVERE PAIN

0	1	2	3	4	5	6	7	8	9	10

SUSPECTED TRIGGERS
-
-
-
-

SYMPTOMS

RELIEF MEASURES

NOTES

CHRONIC PAIN ASSESSMENT

DATE		DAY	
TIME STARTED		TIME ENDED	
TOTAL DURATION			

Mark the location of the pain ←

LENGTH OF TIME EXPERIENCING THE PAIN?

< 6 Months		6-12 Months	
1-3 Years		3 Years +	

TYPE OF PAIN

Indescribable		Stabbing		Sharp	
Burning		Aching		Prickly	
Numb		Tingling/ Pins & Needles			
Other					

EXTERNAL ENVIROMENTAL FACTORS

Sun/ Heat		Cold		Windy	
Rain		Aching		Cloudy	
Other					

PAIN SCALE
NO PAIN ⟶ SEVERE PAIN

0	1	2	3	4	5	6	7	8	9	10

SUSPECTED TRIGGERS
-
-
-
-

-
-
-
-

SYMPTOMS

RELIEF MEASURES

NOTES

CHRONIC PAIN ASSESSMENT

DATE		DAY	
TIME STARTED		**TIME ENDED**	
TOTAL DURATION			

Mark the location of the pain

LENGTH OF TIME EXPERIENCING THE PAIN?

< 6 Months		6-12 Months	
1-3 Years		3 Years +	

TYPE OF PAIN

Indescribable		Stabbing		Sharp	
Burning		Aching		Prickly	
Numb		Tingling/ Pins & Needles			
Other					

EXTERNAL ENVIROMENTAL FACTORS

Sun/ Heat		Cold		Windy	
Rain		Aching		Cloudy	
Other					

PAIN SCALE
NO PAIN ⟶ SEVERE PAIN

0	1	2	3	4	5	6	7	8	9	10

SUSPECTED TRIGGERS
-
-
-
-

SYMPTOMS

RELIEF MEASURES

NOTES

CHRONIC PAIN ASSESSMENT

DATE		DAY	
TIME STARTED		TIME ENDED	
TOTAL DURATION			

← Mark the location of the pain

LENGTH OF TIME EXPERIENCING THE PAIN?

< 6 Months		6-12 Months	
1-3 Years		3 Years +	

TYPE OF PAIN

Indescribable		Stabbing		Sharp	
Burning		Aching		Prickly	
Numb		Tingling/ Pins & Needles			
Other					

EXTERNAL ENVIROMENTAL FACTORS

Sun/ Heat		Cold		Windy	
Rain		Aching		Cloudy	
Other					

PAIN SCALE
NO PAIN ──────────────────────→ SEVERE PAIN

0	1	2	3	4	5	6	7	8	9	10

SUSPECTED TRIGGERS
-
-
-
-

SYMPTOMS

RELIEF MEASURES

NOTES

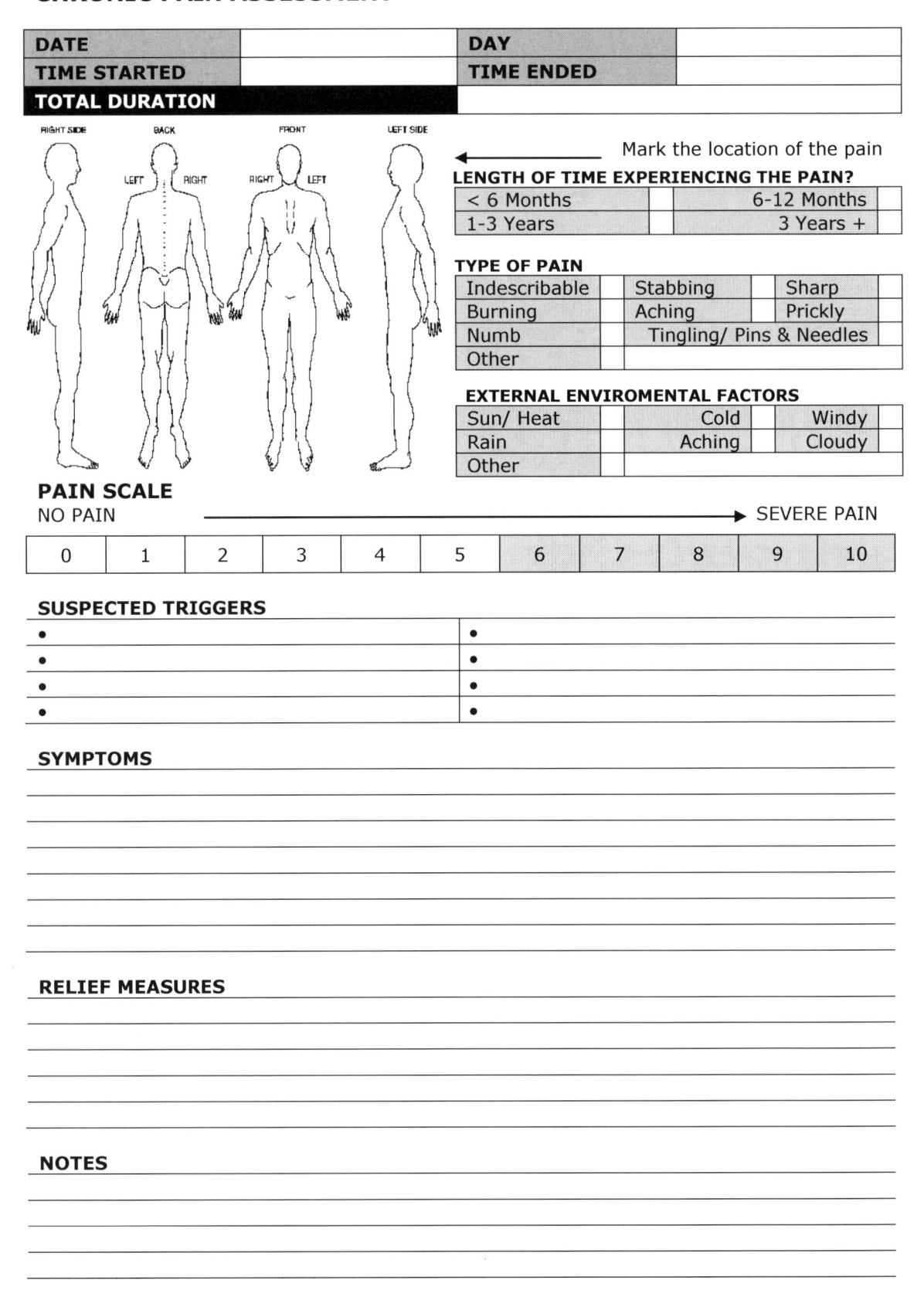

CHRONIC PAIN ASSESSMENT

DATE		DAY	
TIME STARTED		TIME ENDED	
TOTAL DURATION			

← Mark the location of the pain

LENGTH OF TIME EXPERIENCING THE PAIN?

< 6 Months		6-12 Months	
1-3 Years		3 Years +	

TYPE OF PAIN

Indescribable		Stabbing		Sharp	
Burning		Aching		Prickly	
Numb		Tingling/ Pins & Needles			
Other					

EXTERNAL ENVIROMENTAL FACTORS

Sun/ Heat		Cold		Windy	
Rain		Aching		Cloudy	
Other					

PAIN SCALE
NO PAIN → SEVERE PAIN

0	1	2	3	4	5	6	7	8	9	10

SUSPECTED TRIGGERS
-
-
-
-

SYMPTOMS

RELIEF MEASURES

NOTES

CHRONIC PAIN ASSESSMENT

DATE		DAY	
TIME STARTED		TIME ENDED	
TOTAL DURATION			

Mark the location of the pain

LENGTH OF TIME EXPERIENCING THE PAIN?

< 6 Months		6-12 Months	
1-3 Years		3 Years +	

TYPE OF PAIN

Indescribable		Stabbing		Sharp	
Burning		Aching		Prickly	
Numb		Tingling/ Pins & Needles			
Other					

EXTERNAL ENVIROMENTAL FACTORS

Sun/ Heat		Cold		Windy	
Rain		Aching		Cloudy	
Other					

PAIN SCALE
NO PAIN ──────────────────────→ SEVERE PAIN

0	1	2	3	4	5	6	7	8	9	10

SUSPECTED TRIGGERS

-
-
-
-

-
-
-
-

SYMPTOMS

RELIEF MEASURES

NOTES

CHRONIC PAIN ASSESSMENT

DATE		DAY	
TIME STARTED		TIME ENDED	
TOTAL DURATION			

RIGHT SIDE | BACK | FRONT | LEFT SIDE

← Mark the location of the pain

LENGTH OF TIME EXPERIENCING THE PAIN?

< 6 Months		6-12 Months	
1-3 Years		3 Years +	

TYPE OF PAIN

Indescribable		Stabbing		Sharp	
Burning		Aching		Prickly	
Numb		Tingling/ Pins & Needles			
Other					

EXTERNAL ENVIROMENTAL FACTORS

Sun/ Heat		Cold		Windy	
Rain		Aching		Cloudy	
Other					

PAIN SCALE
NO PAIN ──────────────────→ SEVERE PAIN

0	1	2	3	4	5	6	7	8	9	10

SUSPECTED TRIGGERS
-
-
-
-
-
-
-
-

SYMPTOMS

RELIEF MEASURES

NOTES

CHRONIC PAIN ASSESSMENT

DATE		DAY	
TIME STARTED		TIME ENDED	
TOTAL DURATION			

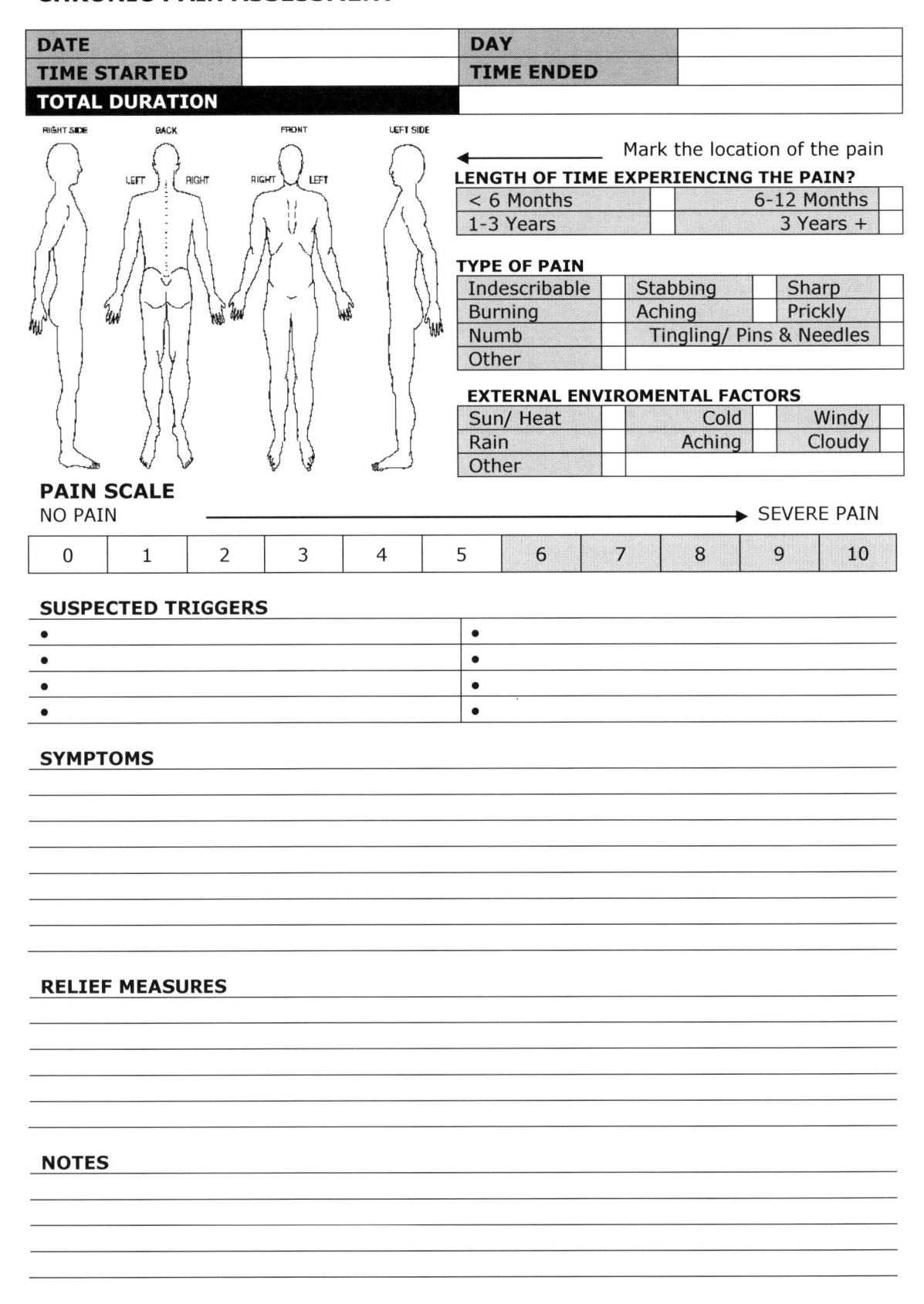

Mark the location of the pain

LENGTH OF TIME EXPERIENCING THE PAIN?

< 6 Months		6-12 Months	
1-3 Years		3 Years +	

TYPE OF PAIN

Indescribable		Stabbing		Sharp	
Burning		Aching		Prickly	
Numb		Tingling/ Pins & Needles			
Other					

EXTERNAL ENVIROMENTAL FACTORS

Sun/ Heat		Cold		Windy	
Rain		Aching		Cloudy	
Other					

PAIN SCALE
NO PAIN → SEVERE PAIN

0	1	2	3	4	5	6	7	8	9	10

SUSPECTED TRIGGERS
-
-
-
-

-
-
-
-

SYMPTOMS

RELIEF MEASURES

NOTES

CHRONIC PAIN ASSESSMENT

DATE		DAY	
TIME STARTED		**TIME ENDED**	
TOTAL DURATION			

Mark the location of the pain

LENGTH OF TIME EXPERIENCING THE PAIN?

< 6 Months		6-12 Months	
1-3 Years		3 Years +	

TYPE OF PAIN

Indescribable		Stabbing		Sharp	
Burning		Aching		Prickly	
Numb		Tingling/ Pins & Needles			
Other					

EXTERNAL ENVIROMENTAL FACTORS

Sun/ Heat		Cold		Windy	
Rain		Aching		Cloudy	
Other					

PAIN SCALE
NO PAIN ──────────────────────→ SEVERE PAIN

0	1	2	3	4	5	6	7	8	9	10

SUSPECTED TRIGGERS
-
-
-
-

SYMPTOMS

RELIEF MEASURES

NOTES

CHRONIC PAIN ASSESSMENT

DATE		DAY	
TIME STARTED		TIME ENDED	
TOTAL DURATION			

Mark the location of the pain

LENGTH OF TIME EXPERIENCING THE PAIN?

< 6 Months		6-12 Months	
1-3 Years		3 Years +	

TYPE OF PAIN

Indescribable		Stabbing		Sharp	
Burning		Aching		Prickly	
Numb		Tingling/ Pins & Needles			
Other					

EXTERNAL ENVIROMENTAL FACTORS

Sun/ Heat		Cold		Windy	
Rain		Aching		Cloudy	
Other					

PAIN SCALE
NO PAIN ──────────────────────────────→ SEVERE PAIN

0	1	2	3	4	5	6	7	8	9	10

SUSPECTED TRIGGERS
-
-
-
-

SYMPTOMS

RELIEF MEASURES

NOTES

CHRONIC PAIN ASSESSMENT

DATE		DAY	
TIME STARTED		TIME ENDED	
TOTAL DURATION			

← Mark the location of the pain

LENGTH OF TIME EXPERIENCING THE PAIN?

< 6 Months		6-12 Months	
1-3 Years		3 Years +	

TYPE OF PAIN

Indescribable		Stabbing		Sharp	
Burning		Aching		Prickly	
Numb		Tingling/ Pins & Needles			
Other					

EXTERNAL ENVIROMENTAL FACTORS

Sun/ Heat		Cold		Windy	
Rain		Aching		Cloudy	
Other					

PAIN SCALE
NO PAIN →→→→→→→→→→→→→→→→→→ SEVERE PAIN

0	1	2	3	4	5	6	7	8	9	10

SUSPECTED TRIGGERS
-
-
-
-
-
-
-
-

SYMPTOMS

RELIEF MEASURES

NOTES

CHRONIC PAIN ASSESSMENT

DATE		DAY	
TIME STARTED		TIME ENDED	
TOTAL DURATION			

← Mark the location of the pain

LENGTH OF TIME EXPERIENCING THE PAIN?

< 6 Months		6-12 Months	
1-3 Years		3 Years +	

TYPE OF PAIN

Indescribable		Stabbing		Sharp	
Burning		Aching		Prickly	
Numb		Tingling/ Pins & Needles			
Other					

EXTERNAL ENVIROMENTAL FACTORS

Sun/ Heat		Cold		Windy	
Rain		Aching		Cloudy	
Other					

PAIN SCALE
NO PAIN ⟶ SEVERE PAIN

0	1	2	3	4	5	6	7	8	9	10

SUSPECTED TRIGGERS
-
-
-
-

SYMPTOMS

RELIEF MEASURES

NOTES

CHRONIC PAIN ASSESSMENT

DATE		DAY	
TIME STARTED		**TIME ENDED**	
TOTAL DURATION			

Mark the location of the pain

LENGTH OF TIME EXPERIENCING THE PAIN?

< 6 Months		6-12 Months	
1-3 Years		3 Years +	

TYPE OF PAIN

Indescribable		Stabbing		Sharp	
Burning		Aching		Prickly	
Numb		Tingling/ Pins & Needles			
Other					

EXTERNAL ENVIROMENTAL FACTORS

Sun/ Heat		Cold		Windy	
Rain		Aching		Cloudy	
Other					

PAIN SCALE
NO PAIN ⟶ SEVERE PAIN

0	1	2	3	4	5	6	7	8	9	10

SUSPECTED TRIGGERS
-
-
-
-
-
-
-
-

SYMPTOMS

RELIEF MEASURES

NOTES

CHRONIC PAIN ASSESSMENT

DATE		DAY	
TIME STARTED		TIME ENDED	
TOTAL DURATION			

Mark the location of the pain

LENGTH OF TIME EXPERIENCING THE PAIN?

< 6 Months		6-12 Months	
1-3 Years		3 Years +	

TYPE OF PAIN

Indescribable		Stabbing		Sharp	
Burning		Aching		Prickly	
Numb		Tingling/ Pins & Needles			
Other					

EXTERNAL ENVIROMENTAL FACTORS

Sun/ Heat		Cold		Windy	
Rain		Aching		Cloudy	
Other					

PAIN SCALE
NO PAIN ⟶ SEVERE PAIN

0	1	2	3	4	5	6	7	8	9	10

SUSPECTED TRIGGERS

-
-
-
-

-
-
-
-

SYMPTOMS

RELIEF MEASURES

NOTES

CHRONIC PAIN ASSESSMENT

DATE		DAY	
TIME STARTED		TIME ENDED	
TOTAL DURATION			

Mark the location of the pain

LENGTH OF TIME EXPERIENCING THE PAIN?

< 6 Months		6-12 Months	
1-3 Years		3 Years +	

TYPE OF PAIN

Indescribable		Stabbing		Sharp	
Burning		Aching		Prickly	
Numb		Tingling/ Pins & Needles			
Other					

EXTERNAL ENVIROMENTAL FACTORS

Sun/ Heat		Cold		Windy	
Rain		Aching		Cloudy	
Other					

PAIN SCALE
NO PAIN ⟶ SEVERE PAIN

0	1	2	3	4	5	6	7	8	9	10

SUSPECTED TRIGGERS
-
-
-
-

-
-
-
-

SYMPTOMS

RELIEF MEASURES

NOTES

CHRONIC PAIN ASSESSMENT

DATE		DAY	
TIME STARTED		**TIME ENDED**	
TOTAL DURATION			

← Mark the location of the pain

LENGTH OF TIME EXPERIENCING THE PAIN?

< 6 Months		6-12 Months	
1-3 Years		3 Years +	

TYPE OF PAIN

Indescribable		Stabbing		Sharp	
Burning		Aching		Prickly	
Numb		Tingling/ Pins & Needles			
Other					

EXTERNAL ENVIROMENTAL FACTORS

Sun/ Heat		Cold		Windy	
Rain		Aching		Cloudy	
Other					

PAIN SCALE
NO PAIN ⟶ SEVERE PAIN

0	1	2	3	4	5	6	7	8	9	10

SUSPECTED TRIGGERS

-
-
-
-

-
-
-
-

SYMPTOMS

RELIEF MEASURES

NOTES

CHRONIC PAIN ASSESSMENT

DATE		DAY	
TIME STARTED		TIME ENDED	
TOTAL DURATION			

← Mark the location of the pain

LENGTH OF TIME EXPERIENCING THE PAIN?

| < 6 Months | | 6-12 Months | |
| 1-3 Years | | 3 Years + | |

TYPE OF PAIN

Indescribable	Stabbing	Sharp
Burning	Aching	Prickly
Numb	Tingling/ Pins & Needles	
Other		

EXTERNAL ENVIROMENTAL FACTORS

Sun/ Heat		Cold		Windy	
Rain		Aching		Cloudy	
Other					

PAIN SCALE
NO PAIN ──────────────────→ SEVERE PAIN

| 0 | 1 | 2 | 3 | 4 | 5 | 6 | 7 | 8 | 9 | 10 |

SUSPECTED TRIGGERS
-
-
-
-

-
-
-
-

SYMPTOMS

RELIEF MEASURES

NOTES

CHRONIC PAIN ASSESSMENT

DATE		DAY	
TIME STARTED		TIME ENDED	
TOTAL DURATION			

← Mark the location of the pain

LENGTH OF TIME EXPERIENCING THE PAIN?

< 6 Months		6-12 Months	
1-3 Years		3 Years +	

TYPE OF PAIN

Indescribable		Stabbing		Sharp	
Burning		Aching		Prickly	
Numb		Tingling/ Pins & Needles			
Other					

EXTERNAL ENVIROMENTAL FACTORS

Sun/ Heat		Cold		Windy	
Rain		Aching		Cloudy	
Other					

PAIN SCALE
NO PAIN ⟶ SEVERE PAIN

0	1	2	3	4	5	6	7	8	9	10

SUSPECTED TRIGGERS

-
-
-
-

-
-
-
-

SYMPTOMS

RELIEF MEASURES

NOTES

CHRONIC PAIN ASSESSMENT

DATE		DAY	
TIME STARTED		TIME ENDED	
TOTAL DURATION			

Mark the location of the pain

LENGTH OF TIME EXPERIENCING THE PAIN?

< 6 Months		6-12 Months	
1-3 Years		3 Years +	

TYPE OF PAIN

Indescribable	Stabbing	Sharp
Burning	Aching	Prickly
Numb	Tingling/ Pins & Needles	
Other		

EXTERNAL ENVIROMENTAL FACTORS

Sun/ Heat	Cold	Windy
Rain	Aching	Cloudy
Other		

PAIN SCALE
NO PAIN → SEVERE PAIN

0	1	2	3	4	5	6	7	8	9	10

SUSPECTED TRIGGERS
-
-
-
-

-
-
-
-

SYMPTOMS

RELIEF MEASURES

NOTES

CHRONIC PAIN ASSESSMENT

DATE		DAY	
TIME STARTED		TIME ENDED	
TOTAL DURATION			

Mark the location of the pain

LENGTH OF TIME EXPERIENCING THE PAIN?
< 6 Months		6-12 Months	
1-3 Years		3 Years +	

TYPE OF PAIN
Indescribable		Stabbing		Sharp	
Burning		Aching		Prickly	
Numb		Tingling/ Pins & Needles			
Other					

EXTERNAL ENVIROMENTAL FACTORS
Sun/ Heat		Cold		Windy	
Rain		Aching		Cloudy	
Other					

PAIN SCALE
NO PAIN ⟶ SEVERE PAIN

0	1	2	3	4	5	6	7	8	9	10

SUSPECTED TRIGGERS
-
-
-
-

SYMPTOMS

RELIEF MEASURES

NOTES

CHRONIC PAIN ASSESSMENT

DATE		DAY	
TIME STARTED		TIME ENDED	
TOTAL DURATION			

Mark the location of the pain

LENGTH OF TIME EXPERIENCING THE PAIN?

< 6 Months		6-12 Months	
1-3 Years		3 Years +	

TYPE OF PAIN

Indescribable		Stabbing		Sharp	
Burning		Aching		Prickly	
Numb		Tingling/ Pins & Needles			
Other					

EXTERNAL ENVIROMENTAL FACTORS

Sun/ Heat		Cold		Windy	
Rain		Aching		Cloudy	
Other					

PAIN SCALE

NO PAIN → SEVERE PAIN

0	1	2	3	4	5	6	7	8	9	10

SUSPECTED TRIGGERS

-
-
-
-

-
-
-
-

SYMPTOMS

RELIEF MEASURES

NOTES

CHRONIC PAIN ASSESSMENT

DATE		DAY	
TIME STARTED		TIME ENDED	
TOTAL DURATION			

← Mark the location of the pain

LENGTH OF TIME EXPERIENCING THE PAIN?

< 6 Months		6-12 Months	
1-3 Years		3 Years +	

TYPE OF PAIN

Indescribable		Stabbing		Sharp	
Burning		Aching		Prickly	
Numb		Tingling/ Pins & Needles	
Other					

EXTERNAL ENVIROMENTAL FACTORS

Sun/ Heat		Cold		Windy	
Rain		Aching		Cloudy	
Other					

PAIN SCALE
NO PAIN ⟶ SEVERE PAIN

| 0 | 1 | 2 | 3 | 4 | 5 | 6 | 7 | 8 | 9 | 10 |

SUSPECTED TRIGGERS
-
-
-
-

-
-
-
-

SYMPTOMS

RELIEF MEASURES

NOTES

CHRONIC PAIN ASSESSMENT

DATE		DAY	
TIME STARTED		TIME ENDED	
TOTAL DURATION			

Mark the location of the pain

LENGTH OF TIME EXPERIENCING THE PAIN?

< 6 Months		6-12 Months	
1-3 Years		3 Years +	

TYPE OF PAIN

Indescribable	Stabbing	Sharp
Burning	Aching	Prickly
Numb	Tingling/ Pins & Needles	
Other		

EXTERNAL ENVIROMENTAL FACTORS

Sun/ Heat	Cold	Windy
Rain	Aching	Cloudy
Other		

PAIN SCALE
NO PAIN ⟶ SEVERE PAIN

0	1	2	3	4	5	6	7	8	9	10

SUSPECTED TRIGGERS
-
-
-
-

SYMPTOMS

RELIEF MEASURES

NOTES

CHRONIC PAIN ASSESSMENT

DATE		DAY	
TIME STARTED		TIME ENDED	
TOTAL DURATION			

RIGHT SIDE BACK FRONT LEFT SIDE

← Mark the location of the pain

LENGTH OF TIME EXPERIENCING THE PAIN?

< 6 Months		6-12 Months	
1-3 Years		3 Years +	

TYPE OF PAIN

Indescribable		Stabbing		Sharp	
Burning		Aching		Prickly	
Numb		Tingling/ Pins & Needles			
Other					

EXTERNAL ENVIROMENTAL FACTORS

Sun/ Heat		Cold		Windy	
Rain		Aching		Cloudy	
Other					

PAIN SCALE
NO PAIN ──────────────────→ SEVERE PAIN

0	1	2	3	4	5	6	7	8	9	10

SUSPECTED TRIGGERS

-
-
-
-

-
-
-
-

SYMPTOMS

RELIEF MEASURES

NOTES

CHRONIC PAIN ASSESSMENT

DATE		DAY	
TIME STARTED		TIME ENDED	
TOTAL DURATION			

← Mark the location of the pain

LENGTH OF TIME EXPERIENCING THE PAIN?

< 6 Months		6-12 Months	
1-3 Years		3 Years +	

TYPE OF PAIN

Indescribable		Stabbing		Sharp	
Burning		Aching		Prickly	
Numb		Tingling/ Pins & Needles			
Other					

EXTERNAL ENVIRONMENTAL FACTORS

Sun/ Heat		Cold		Windy	
Rain		Aching		Cloudy	
Other					

PAIN SCALE

NO PAIN ──────────────────→ SEVERE PAIN

0	1	2	3	4	5	6	7	8	9	10

SUSPECTED TRIGGERS

-
-
-
-

-
-
-
-

SYMPTOMS

RELIEF MEASURES

NOTES

CHRONIC PAIN ASSESSMENT

DATE		DAY	
TIME STARTED		TIME ENDED	
TOTAL DURATION			

← Mark the location of the pain

LENGTH OF TIME EXPERIENCING THE PAIN?

< 6 Months		6-12 Months	
1-3 Years		3 Years +	

TYPE OF PAIN

Indescribable		Stabbing		Sharp	
Burning		Aching		Prickly	
Numb		Tingling/ Pins & Needles			
Other					

EXTERNAL ENVIROMENTAL FACTORS

Sun/ Heat		Cold		Windy	
Rain		Aching		Cloudy	
Other					

PAIN SCALE
NO PAIN ⟶ SEVERE PAIN

0	1	2	3	4	5	6	7	8	9	10

SUSPECTED TRIGGERS
-
-
-
-

-
-
-
-

SYMPTOMS

RELIEF MEASURES

NOTES

CHRONIC PAIN ASSESSMENT

DATE		DAY	
TIME STARTED		TIME ENDED	
TOTAL DURATION			

Mark the location of the pain

LENGTH OF TIME EXPERIENCING THE PAIN?

< 6 Months		6-12 Months	
1-3 Years		3 Years +	

TYPE OF PAIN

Indescribable		Stabbing		Sharp	
Burning		Aching		Prickly	
Numb		Tingling/ Pins & Needles			
Other					

EXTERNAL ENVIROMENTAL FACTORS

Sun/ Heat		Cold		Windy	
Rain		Aching		Cloudy	
Other					

PAIN SCALE
NO PAIN ──────────────────────► SEVERE PAIN

0	1	2	3	4	5	6	7	8	9	10

SUSPECTED TRIGGERS
-
-
-
-
-
-
-
-

SYMPTOMS

RELIEF MEASURES

NOTES

CHRONIC PAIN ASSESSMENT

DATE		DAY	
TIME STARTED		TIME ENDED	
TOTAL DURATION			

Mark the location of the pain

LENGTH OF TIME EXPERIENCING THE PAIN?

< 6 Months		6-12 Months	
1-3 Years		3 Years +	

TYPE OF PAIN

Indescribable		Stabbing		Sharp	
Burning		Aching		Prickly	
Numb		Tingling/ Pins & Needles			
Other					

EXTERNAL ENVIROMENTAL FACTORS

Sun/ Heat		Cold		Windy	
Rain		Aching		Cloudy	
Other					

PAIN SCALE
NO PAIN ⟶ SEVERE PAIN

0	1	2	3	4	5	6	7	8	9	10

SUSPECTED TRIGGERS

-
-
-
-

-
-
-
-

SYMPTOMS

RELIEF MEASURES

NOTES

CHRONIC PAIN ASSESSMENT

DATE		DAY	
TIME STARTED		TIME ENDED	
TOTAL DURATION			

Mark the location of the pain

LENGTH OF TIME EXPERIENCING THE PAIN?

< 6 Months		6-12 Months	
1-3 Years		3 Years +	

TYPE OF PAIN

Indescribable		Stabbing		Sharp	
Burning		Aching		Prickly	
Numb		Tingling/ Pins & Needles			
Other					

EXTERNAL ENVIROMENTAL FACTORS

Sun/ Heat		Cold		Windy	
Rain		Aching		Cloudy	
Other					

PAIN SCALE
NO PAIN → SEVERE PAIN

0	1	2	3	4	5	6	7	8	9	10

SUSPECTED TRIGGERS
-
-
-
-

SYMPTOMS

RELIEF MEASURES

NOTES

CHRONIC PAIN ASSESSMENT

DATE		DAY	
TIME STARTED		TIME ENDED	
TOTAL DURATION			

RIGHT SIDE — BACK (LEFT / RIGHT) — FRONT (RIGHT / LEFT) — LEFT SIDE

← Mark the location of the pain

LENGTH OF TIME EXPERIENCING THE PAIN?

< 6 Months		6-12 Months	
1-3 Years		3 Years +	

TYPE OF PAIN

Indescribable		Stabbing		Sharp	
Burning		Aching		Prickly	
Numb		Tingling/ Pins & Needles			
Other					

EXTERNAL ENVIROMENTAL FACTORS

Sun/ Heat		Cold		Windy	
Rain		Aching		Cloudy	
Other					

PAIN SCALE
NO PAIN ────────────────────────→ SEVERE PAIN

0	1	2	3	4	5	6	7	8	9	10

SUSPECTED TRIGGERS

-
-
-
-

-
-
-
-

SYMPTOMS

RELIEF MEASURES

NOTES

CHRONIC PAIN ASSESSMENT

DATE		DAY	
TIME STARTED		TIME ENDED	
TOTAL DURATION			

← Mark the location of the pain

LENGTH OF TIME EXPERIENCING THE PAIN?

< 6 Months		6-12 Months	
1-3 Years		3 Years +	

TYPE OF PAIN

Indescribable	Stabbing	Sharp
Burning	Aching	Prickly
Numb	Tingling/ Pins & Needles	
Other		

EXTERNAL ENVIROMENTAL FACTORS

Sun/ Heat	Cold	Windy
Rain	Aching	Cloudy
Other		

PAIN SCALE
NO PAIN ⟶ SEVERE PAIN

| 0 | 1 | 2 | 3 | 4 | 5 | 6 | 7 | 8 | 9 | 10 |

SUSPECTED TRIGGERS
-
-
-
-

-
-
-
-

SYMPTOMS

RELIEF MEASURES

NOTES

CHRONIC PAIN ASSESSMENT

DATE		DAY	
TIME STARTED		TIME ENDED	
TOTAL DURATION			

RIGHT SIDE BACK FRONT LEFT SIDE
LEFT RIGHT RIGHT LEFT

← Mark the location of the pain

LENGTH OF TIME EXPERIENCING THE PAIN?

< 6 Months		6-12 Months	
1-3 Years		3 Years +	

TYPE OF PAIN

Indescribable		Stabbing		Sharp	
Burning		Aching		Prickly	
Numb		Tingling/ Pins & Needles			
Other					

EXTERNAL ENVIROMENTAL FACTORS

Sun/ Heat		Cold		Windy	
Rain		Aching		Cloudy	
Other					

PAIN SCALE
NO PAIN ——————————————→ SEVERE PAIN

0	1	2	3	4	5	6	7	8	9	10

SUSPECTED TRIGGERS
-
-
-
-

-
-
-
-

SYMPTOMS

RELIEF MEASURES

NOTES

CHRONIC PAIN ASSESSMENT

DATE		DAY	
TIME STARTED		TIME ENDED	
TOTAL DURATION			

Mark the location of the pain

LENGTH OF TIME EXPERIENCING THE PAIN?

< 6 Months		6-12 Months	
1-3 Years		3 Years +	

TYPE OF PAIN

Indescribable		Stabbing		Sharp	
Burning		Aching		Prickly	
Numb		Tingling/ Pins & Needles			
Other					

EXTERNAL ENVIROMENTAL FACTORS

Sun/ Heat		Cold		Windy	
Rain		Aching		Cloudy	
Other					

PAIN SCALE

NO PAIN ──────────────────────────────→ SEVERE PAIN

0	1	2	3	4	5	6	7	8	9	10

SUSPECTED TRIGGERS

-
-
-
-

-
-
-
-

SYMPTOMS

RELIEF MEASURES

NOTES

TREATMENT HISTORY- PRESCRIPTION MEDICATION

MEDICATION NAME	DATE STARTED	START DOSE	DATE ENDED	END DOSE

RESULT & NOTES	

MEDICATION NAME	DATE STARTED	START DOSE	DATE ENDED	END DOSE

RESULT & NOTES	

MEDICATION NAME	DATE STARTED	START DOSE	DATE ENDED	END DOSE

RESULT & NOTES	

MEDICATION NAME	DATE STARTED	START DOSE	DATE ENDED	END DOSE

RESULT & NOTES	

MEDICATION NAME	DATE STARTED	START DOSE	DATE ENDED	END DOSE

RESULT & NOTES	

MEDICATION NAME	DATE STARTED	START DOSE	DATE ENDED	END DOSE

RESULT & NOTES	

MEDICATION NAME	DATE STARTED	START DOSE	DATE ENDED	END DOSE

RESULT & NOTES	

TREATMENT HISTORY- NON PRESCRIPTION

DESCRIPTION	DATE	RESULTS & NOTES

DESCRIPTION	DATE	RESULTS & NOTES

DESCRIPTION	DATE	RESULTS & NOTES

DESCRIPTION	DATE	RESULTS & NOTES

DESCRIPTION	DATE	RESULTS & NOTES

DESCRIPTION	DATE	RESULTS & NOTES

DESCRIPTION	DATE	RESULTS & NOTES

DESCRIPTION	DATE	RESULTS & NOTES

DESCRIPTION	DATE	RESULTS & NOTES

DESCRIPTION	DATE	RESULTS & NOTES

DESCRIPTION	DATE	RESULTS & NOTES

DESCRIPTION	DATE	RESULTS & NOTES

DESCRIPTION	DATE	RESULTS & NOTES

DESCRIPTION	DATE	RESULTS & NOTES

TREATMENT HISTORY - PRESCRIPTION MEDICATION

MEDICATION NAME	DATE STARTED	START DOSE	DATE ENDED	END DOSE

RESULT & NOTES	

MEDICATION NAME	DATE STARTED	START DOSE	DATE ENDED	END DOSE

RESULT & NOTES	

MEDICATION NAME	DATE STARTED	START DOSE	DATE ENDED	END DOSE

RESULT & NOTES	

MEDICATION NAME	DATE STARTED	START DOSE	DATE ENDED	END DOSE

RESULT & NOTES	

MEDICATION NAME	DATE STARTED	START DOSE	DATE ENDED	END DOSE

RESULT & NOTES	

MEDICATION NAME	DATE STARTED	START DOSE	DATE ENDED	END DOSE

RESULT & NOTES	

MEDICATION NAME	DATE STARTED	START DOSE	DATE ENDED	END DOSE

RESULT & NOTES	

TREATMENT HISTORY- NON PRESCRIPTION

DESCRIPTION	DATE	RESULTS & NOTES

DESCRIPTION	DATE	RESULTS & NOTES

DESCRIPTION	DATE	RESULTS & NOTES

DESCRIPTION	DATE	RESULTS & NOTES

DESCRIPTION	DATE	RESULTS & NOTES

DESCRIPTION	DATE	RESULTS & NOTES

DESCRIPTION	DATE	RESULTS & NOTES

DESCRIPTION	DATE	RESULTS & NOTES

DESCRIPTION	DATE	RESULTS & NOTES

DESCRIPTION	DATE	RESULTS & NOTES

DESCRIPTION	DATE	RESULTS & NOTES

DESCRIPTION	DATE	RESULTS & NOTES

DESCRIPTION	DATE	RESULTS & NOTES

DESCRIPTION	DATE	RESULTS & NOTES

DOCTORS/ CLINIC APPOINTMENTS

DATE	TIME	WITH	REASON

NOTES/ RESULT

DATE	TIME	WITH	REASON

NOTES/ RESULT

DATE	TIME	WITH	REASON

NOTES/ RESULT

DATE	TIME	WITH	REASON

NOTES/ RESULT

DATE	TIME	WITH	REASON

NOTES/ RESULT

DOCTORS/ CLINIC APPOINTMENTS

DATE	TIME	WITH	REASON

NOTES/ RESULT

DATE	TIME	WITH	REASON

NOTES/ RESULT

DATE	TIME	WITH	REASON

NOTES/ RESULT

DATE	TIME	WITH	REASON

NOTES/ RESULT

DATE	TIME	WITH	REASON

NOTES/ RESULT

DOCTORS/ CLINIC APPOINTMENTS

DATE	TIME	WITH	REASON

NOTES/ RESULT

DATE	TIME	WITH	REASON

NOTES/ RESULT

DATE	TIME	WITH	REASON

NOTES/ RESULT

DATE	TIME	WITH	REASON

NOTES/ RESULT

DATE	TIME	WITH	REASON

NOTES/ RESULT

DOCTORS/ CLINIC APPOINTMENTS

DATE	TIME	WITH	REASON

NOTES/ RESULT

_____
_____
_____

DATE	TIME	WITH	REASON

NOTES/ RESULT

_____
_____
_____

DATE	TIME	WITH	REASON

NOTES/ RESULT

_____
_____
_____

DATE	TIME	WITH	REASON

NOTES/ RESULT

_____
_____
_____

DATE	TIME	WITH	REASON

NOTES/ RESULT

_____
_____
_____

DOCTORS/ CLINIC APPOINTMENTS

DATE	TIME	WITH	REASON

NOTES/ RESULT

DATE	TIME	WITH	REASON

NOTES/ RESULT

DATE	TIME	WITH	REASON

NOTES/ RESULT

DATE	TIME	WITH	REASON

NOTES/ RESULT

DATE	TIME	WITH	REASON

NOTES/ RESULT

DOCTORS/ CLINIC APPOINTMENTS

DATE	TIME	WITH	REASON

NOTES/ RESULT

DATE	TIME	WITH	REASON

NOTES/ RESULT

DATE	TIME	WITH	REASON

NOTES/ RESULT

DATE	TIME	WITH	REASON

NOTES/ RESULT

DATE	TIME	WITH	REASON

NOTES/ RESULT

NOTES

NOTES

NOTES

NOTES

NOTES

Printed in Great Britain
by Amazon